Blessings at Midnight

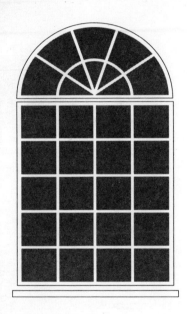

A true story
of hope
when things
seemed hopeless

Kay Kuzma

Pacific Press® Publishing Association
Nampa, Idaho
Oshawa, Ontario, Canada

Edited by Jerry D. Thomas
Cover photo by Stan Sinclair
Designed by Dennis Ferree

Copyright©1998 by
Pacific Press® Publishing Association
Printed in the United States of America
All Rights Reserved

Kuzma, Kay
    Blessings at midnight : a true story of hope when things
seemed hopeless /Kay Kuzma.
        p.   cm.
    ISBN 0-8163-1685-6
    1. Kuzma, Jan W.—Health. 2. Cerebrovascular disease—
Patients-United States—Biography. 3. Cerebrovascular
disease—Religious aspects—Christianity. I. Title.
RC388.5.K89   1998
362.1′9681—dc21
[b]   98-29405
                                                        CIP

98 99 00 01 02 • 5 4 3 2 1

Dedication

Dedicated to my loving husband, Jan, my travel companion through the unexpected challenges of life, who has held on to hope in the darkest hours.

This should be my husband's book. I am weak in hope, with emotions that roll and tumble as waves crash over me. But he is strong. Throughout our thirty-five years together, Jan has kept the blanket of hope tucked in tightly around us, regardless of the circumstances.

His hope is the buoy that holds my head above churning water.

His hope is the rudder that keeps us pointed toward God's harbor when the currents of despair threaten to sweep me away.

His hope is the oil that soothes my anxious heart and quiets my troubled mind.

And so I dedicate this book to him.

Contents

Acknowledgments

To those who were there to offer hope in my darkest hours . . .

To my church family and friends who came to the waiting room to pray for all I held dear when lives were hanging in the balance. And to the hundreds who could not come but called, wrote, and lifted us up in prayer. And to the elders who anointed my husband and prayed—and were part of the miracle. Especially, I want to thank Kari and Jeff St. Clair, Betty Hoehn, Hans Diehl, Elden Chalmers, Charlene and Chuck Robertson, Dave and Joanie Everts, John and Dona Reinhold, and Dianne and Gary Affolter who by their presence and encouragement gave us hope to face an uncertain future.

And to God, who revealed in the middle of Lamentations, the book of weeping, these incredible words . . .

"Yet there is one ray of **hope***: his compassion never ends"* (Lam. 3:21, TLB).

*B*ut I will hope continually,
And will praise You yet more and more.
My mouth shall tell of Your righteousness
And Your salvation all the day,
For I do not know their limits

(Ps. 71:14, 15, NKJV).

Introduction

I never set out to write a book about hope.

I much prefer living on a sunlit mountaintop where the view is great—where it's easy to believe, easy to trust, and easy to see what's ahead. On the mountaintop, there's not much need for hope. I much prefer praise, thanksgiving, joy, peace, and contentment. Those are the emotions I cherish.

You see, one should not write about that which one hasn't experienced, and living on the mountaintop seemed much more appealing to me than walking through the valley of the shadow of death where one discovers the incredible power of hope. Hope comes alive in the down times. Hope is fueled in the fire of troubles and trials—if you will give it the prayer power it needs to burn. But who wants the troubles and trials? I certainly didn't.

Just as the stars are brightest on the darkest nights, so is hope. But the dark times in life are not something one looks forward to. Hurt, pain, death, disease, accidents, trials, hardships, and disappointments are the stuff out of which hope is born. But the accompanying pain—like labor pain—isn't something for which one wishes. So for many, hope is merely a word without much meaning.

And then it happens to you! Your husband has a massive stroke; the doctor says you can count the months you have to live on your fingers; your baby is born with brain damage or a birth defect; the accident turns your teenager into a quadriplegic. You learn there's no remedy for your pain, and you're just going to have to live with it; your job is snatched away, and you find yourself on food stamps. You're falsely accused; you're dragged into a lawsuit against your will; your investments sour, and your life savings are drained; or you're rejected by the people you thought were friends. Your husband leaves you, your wife dies, your children blame you, your parents criticize you—and you don't think you can go on another day.

When that happens, you are about to experience the most incredible miracle that God can work in the human heart—the miracle of hope. It's the miracle of hope that wells up in your being. It gives you the courage to hold on, to look up, and to become with God in the valley of life more than you could ever become by yourself on the mountaintop.

I know! My husband, Jan, and I have experienced it! This is our story since that fateful Thursday, in the winter of 1996 when life as we had known it came to a screeching halt—and our life of hope began. But more than that, this is the story of Jan's life circumstances that chiseled into his being a remarkable trust in God that not even a major strike against him could shake.

If you feel you've got a strike or two against you, it is our prayer that you will find the hope that we did in God's promise . . .

"I know the plans I have for you, says the Lord. They are plans for good and not for evil, to give you a future and a hope" (Jer. 29:11, TLB).

. . . and experience blessings even in the darkness of midnight.

CHAPTER
One

When the Good Life Turns Bad

On Thursday, February 8, 1996, my husband, Jan, and I had an active day at our desks in our beautiful Tennessee country home. That morning, Jan had finished another draft of his book on lifestyle practices, and after getting it in the mail to his co-writer, he spent the rest of his day reading some financial newsletters and sorting through some junk mail. All over the floor he had piles of things to do. I was busy writing radio scripts and answering messages. We had spent the last week on a speaking trip in Florida and were leaving in twelve days for California. And, like always, there was too much to do.

About eleven o'clock that morning, I looked at my calendar and noticed that an Advent Home board meeting was scheduled for 6:30 that evening. I always tried to go if I was in town because I really cared about the rehabilitation school for boys in Calhoun, Tennessee, that Blondel and Gloria Senior operated. But I just didn't feel like going. I could have begged off by saying I had too much to do trying administering the Family Matters organization and keeping up an aggressive writing schedule, but that wasn't true this time—I could have found the time if I had wanted to. So I dialed and left a disjointed message, "I won't be coming to the board meeting tonight, I have ... I need to ... I don't have the ... I just don't feel like coming."

That's why I was home at 6:30 that evening when Jan finally left his office, walked down the hall past mine, and reminded me that it was suppertime.

Usually we eat at 6:30, watch the evening news together, and are back at our evening duties a little after seven. But just as I was about to hit the save function on my computer and put it to sleep, I got a long-distance call. Jan and I both work out of our home and get business calls at all hours of the day and night, so mealtime interruptions are something we have grown to reluctantly accept. I waved him on to the kitchen and mouthed the message that I would come as soon as I was finished.

He began supper preparations and started eating. I finally came about 6:50, throwing our evening routine a little late. A broken pipe meant that Jan was planning to spend some time that evening vacuuming water off the basement floor. But because I was late, Jan was still in the kitchen at 7:20. And I was there with him, instead of being back at my computer when it happened. That dreaded killer called STROKE, struck!

Jan's heart had an atrial septile defect. The hole that was supposed to close at birth, didn't. From the time he was a little boy, he knew he had an irregular heartbeat. But since he was an avid soccer player as a teen, enjoyed tennis through college, hiked, swam, and carried on a good daily exercise program, no one suspected anything more serious.

But when Jan was fifty-four, during a routine physical examination at Loma Linda University, Dr. Raymond Herber noticed an enlarged vein in his neck and referred him to Dr. Ken Jutzy, a cardiologist, who discovered the atrial septile defect. It was repaired with an experimental procedure, but even with repeated shocks to his heart, the irregular beat continued, which put him at risk for the formation of blood clots. The anti-coagulant, Coumidin (which has been used as a rat poison), was the answer. He had to keep his blood "thin" so a clot wouldn't form.

But in the five years since that time, things had changed. Jan had developed an "anticancer" diet of broccoli, Brussels sprouts, cabbage, greens, and soy. The more he learned about the protective benefits of these foods, the more he ate, never realizing that the additional Vitamin K (a coagulant) he was ingesting was counteracting the effects of the Coumidin.

To add to this imbalance, just the week before his stroke, Jan had begun to feel that the Coumidin he was taking was causing him to feel lethargic. Since he had always avoided as many medications as possible, he decided to cut back a little to see if he wouldn't feel better. A few days later, after consulting with a physician in Florida who said, "If you don't keep up your dosage, I'm afraid you'll have a stroke," he had resumed taking his regular amount. But alas, the die was cast. The clot formed and was released like a bomb, exploding in his brain that fateful night in February.

Those hours were permanently etched into my memory by the emotional trauma I experienced. About 7:20, Jan was telling me, as he poured himself a glass of orange juice, about the Caribbean plane carrying more than two hundred German tourists that had crashed in shark-infested waters. Being European, he prefers to take the refrigerated chill off his drink. But just as he started to put the glass into the microwave, he began to slur his words, stuttering "sha, sha, shark infest, fest, fested" and I noticed the left side of his face begin to quiver and drop. I asked sharply, "Honey, are you OK?"

He said, "Yes," and continued trying to bring the glass in his left hand up to the microwave.

I immediately jumped up from the table and shouted, "Jan, I think you're having a stroke." I grabbed his left side, took the glass from his hand, and yelled to Todd, "Todd, come help me, I think Jan is having a stroke." Todd rooms downstairs, but he just happened to be up in our living room watching TV since the floor of his apartment was flooded. Todd jumped up and ran to Jan's other side, and we walked him to a kitchen chair and sat him down, where seconds later, he lost all left-side function and began to drool from the left side of his mouth.

The timing still amazes me: It happened when I was home and still in the kitchen with Jan and when Todd was upstairs to give immediate help. We were right there to grab Jan before he fell. He could have cracked his head on the tile counters or floor. Or if it had happened fifteen minutes later, Jan could have been lying on the cold, wet floor downstairs, unable to move, waiting for help for who knows how long!

The panic that struck me was terrifying. My heart raced, my hands turned clammy, my memory failed—I couldn't think of telephone numbers I routinely called—or the hospital in Chattanooga, where I had determined I would go to if I was ever involved in a medical emergency. I grabbed the phone list of our friends and family. I frantically dialed, hands shaking so badly I could hardly keep my fingers on the numbers I wanted to call. I dialed three of our closest friends and the pastor. No one was home. I had to find out where to take Jan and get the prayer chains started. I finally reached Helen Becker, a friend and nurse, and Helen said, "Call 911 and take him to Memorial in Chattanooga."

As soon as I knew help was on the way, I called our children and Jan's brother and sisters, leaving messages about what had happened and where we'd be. Then I packed—my toothbrush and laptop computer—ready to ride along in the ambulance, not knowing what the future held.

Jan knew the paramedics were coming, but that's the last thing he remembered until he realized he was in the Intensive Care Unit in Memorial. Still, he didn't believe he'd had a stroke.

The eighth was a cold wintry night in Cleveland, Tennessee. Snow was still covering the ground from a recent storm. If Jan's stroke would have happened the night before, I wonder if the paramedics could have made it up our icy drive. I shudder to think of the time delay if they would have had to hike into our place and carry him down to the road on a stretcher.

If one could plan the best time to have a stroke—which one can't—I'd say the timing of Jan's was just about perfect. All I know is that the One who created us, monitors our systems, and knows when our bodies are about to experience a crisis can impress people and alter situations to provide the help we need at those times when a crisis is inevitable. And I believe God was definitely working things out in our case.

Another incredible thing—the medical attendant in the ambulance knew us! He looked at Todd and said, "You look familiar." They had gone to Union College together. He also had read one of my books. It was reassuring to know that Jan was in the hands of a friend. As we pulled out of our drive, the medic was trying to check the pupils of Jan's eyes. Later I was told he had a slight seizure.

The driver and medic were determined to take Jan to Bradley Memorial—our local hospital. They said that was their policy. Jan's condition would be stabilized there, and then he could be moved to the hospital of our choice. I insisted that Jan be immediately taken to Memorial. We would lose valuable time going to the local hospital since it was on the far side of town, but if we would head directly to Chattanooga, it would take only fifteen minutes longer than going to Bradley. I was adamant about this. I knew I had to get him to Memorial! The attendants established radio contact with a Bradley Memorial emergency care doctor, and he pronounced Jan's condition "stabilized" and gave us permission to go directly to Memorial.

It was a good thing, because within a half hour of our arrival, our good friends, Dave and Joanie Everts were there by my side in the emergency waiting room. A half-hour later, having just gotten my message, our pastor, Steve Haley, arrived—with a 103-degree temperature and not feeling exactly on top of the world! Shortly after, another good friend, Lennart Wahlne, arrived. Charlene Robertson, head of the nursing staff at Memorial, got my message when she got home that evening and phoned the emergency room to talk with me. Within minutes Charlene and her husband, Chuck, old college friends of Jan's, were there.

Charlene, knowing the staff, arranged for the emergency physician and the cardiologist assigned to Jan's case to talk immediately with me, while they allowed Pastor Steve to have prayer with Jan. Then he was taken for a CAT scan. As he was being wheeled in, I asked Jan where his cardiac medical records were, and he told me they were on the third or fourth shelf of a horizontal metal file holder in the cabinet above his desk. During this time he didn't initiate conversation, but he could answer when asked a question.

It was during the CAT scan, as Charlene and I watched, that Jan moved his left arm slightly. Then later back in the emergency examining room, I saw him move his left foot a little. At that moment, any slight movement was good news—very good news.

By midnight Jan had been assigned the last available bed in ICU, and I was standing by his side holding his hand, praying for him and telling him what had happened. What I didn't tell him was that none of the physicians held much hope. The word I had gotten from them was, "It was a big one. Massive. And I'm so, so sorry for you."

Dave and Joanie took me home that night, driving down the winding country roads through dense fog, arriving about 1:30 a.m. As I look back over the events of those first few hours, the density of the fog was symbolic of the fog of despair that settled over me as I showered and crawled into bed. I set the alarm to ring early. ICU visiting hours were from 8:00 to 8:30 in the morning, and I determined to be there. But as it turned out, I didn't need an alarm. I tossed and turned, prayed and sobbed, the night away. I was up and packed—not knowing when I would return—way before I needed to leave.

The cardiologist, Dr. Gordon Graham, came by ICU early and consulted with Dr. Sharon Farber, Jan's neurologist, in hushed tones beside his bed. Dr. Farber asked Jan some questions like who he was, what day it was, and who was president. She then asked him to draw a clock and put the numbers on it. Jan thought he passed her "tests" with flying colors, but later she showed me the clock he had drawn with the twelve and six in the right positions but the seven and eight were where the four and five should have been.

Dr. Graham left ICU before relatives were allowed in and stopped to speak with me in the hallway, "I'm so sorry. It's not good. It was dense. Very dense." I still didn't know what "dense" meant. Later I learned that the clot hit a central core area of the right side of Jan's brain, meaning that all the brain cells beyond the point of the clot would likely be damaged or destroyed. Anytime a portion of the brain—for a brief critical period of time—is deprived of the blood that carries oxygen and vital nutrients to it, the affected area fails to function normally and is in danger of dying.

A dense or core stroke, like the one Jan suffered, is something very different from a peripheral one affecting the surface area of the brain where the damaged area is usually less extensive. The CAT scan showed that the blood clot had blocked Jan's right middle cerebral artery, impairing the blood flow to the head of his left caudate nucleus, lenticular nucleus, part of the internal capsule, and his frontal and temporal lobes. With these areas impaired, it would be expected that there could be major devastation and an inability to use the left side of his body. Plus, there was evidence of difficulty with spatial and time perceptions, and analytic thinking. And the doctors feared that the damage would be permanent. The one bright spot was that the CAT scan showed no sign of hemorrhage, which was further evidence that the stroke was caused by a clot from his heart and not a burst blood vessel in the brain.

At this point, although Jan was oblivious to it all, a medical decision had to be made. Since his blood-clotting time (pro-time) was twelve, which was in the normal range rather than between sixteen to eighteen where it should have been, the cardiologist and all the other physicians I talked to, including Jan's brother, George, were concerned that his heart would throw another clot. That would cause more damage— or even death. All said, "Get Warfarin started immediately." Warfarin, like Coumidin, is an anticoagulant but is given intravenously to immediately "thin" the blood, while Coumidin is given orally and reacts more slowly.

Since Jan was admitted as a stroke patient, the primary physician assigned to his case was Dr. Farber, the neurologist, not the cardiologist. And Dr. Farber said No. She felt the risk of throwing another clot was not as great as the risk of hemorrhaging at the already affected site. So for the next twenty-four hours, I sat on pins and needles praying that Dr. Farber was right and Jan's heart wouldn't throw another clot.

When I was finally let in to see Jan on Friday morning, Dr. Farber leveled with me. "Your husband suffered a massive stroke, which has affected his left side, his spatial orientation, and his analytic thinking. He will probably never work again, so I'd suggest that you apply for full disability insurance."

Stunned, I blurted, "But what about all the people who get better? Can't you give me any hope?" Dr. Farber shrugged her shoulders. "One-third get better, one-third stay the same, and one-third get worse," she said.

I was devastated. But I kept it all inside as I leaned over Jan's tubes and kissed him aggressively. He eagerly responded. He might have had a stroke, he might have been a captive in a body that no longer responded to his will, but I

19

wanted him to know he was loved. I kept saying to him, "Precious, we can make it. Together, we can do anything. Already your left arm and leg are moving a little, and your grip is good."

I told him our daughter, Kari, who is a physical therapist, and her husband, Jeff, were on their way from Michigan and that prayer chains had spread throughout the world. Thousands of people were praying for him. And then the half-hour was up, and I was told it was time to go.

Jan slept.

But it would be a long time before I could sleep. Saddled with the unwelcome news of Jan's prognosis, I made my way to the ICU waiting room, crowded with the relatives of cardiac patients. Every thirty minutes or so, a gowned physician would open the door, say a name, people would jump to their feet, and the word given, "Bypass surgery went well. He's in recovery." The joy was spontaneous among those who held vigil. Smiles burst forth.

Those who wait tend to make friends among themselves, but I sat alone with my thoughts. What would happen to us? How would I manage the maintenance of our home if Jan were to get no better? How would I take care of him and keep up my work too? How was all this going to be paid for? What about our future income? I prayed for a miracle for Jan—for us—and then in the midst of my discouragement, the phone rang. "Kuzma," someone shouted.

I took the phone and heard the words, "Kay, it's Hans. I just heard about Jan. Don't listen to the doctors if they tell you Jan won't get better. He can. I know many stroke patients who have worked hard at rehabilitation and today, except for a slight limp or the inability to use a hand, you'd never know."

He went on to tell me about Dexter Yeager who suffered a stroke before the age of fifty but was now one of the most successful businessmen in North Carolina (a multi-millionaire) and a much-sought-after motivational speaker. The only difference between life before the stroke and life now was that he now signs his checks with his left hand.

Hans closed with this admonition, "What Jan needs now from you, Kay, is encouragement. You must give him hope. He's going to need motivation to continue the hard work of rehabilitation. Don't let him get discouraged! God can give you a miracle. Jan can get well."

What a difference in the way I left Jan that morning and when I returned for the noon visitation time! Earlier that day, the negative news had destroyed me. I had nothing to give. I was empty, heavy with a burden I didn't know how I'd carry. Now I was filled with hope, and my positive attitude was contagious. I told Jan all about Hans Diehl's phone call. Hans was his former graduate student who was now directing the Lifestyle Medicine Institute in Loma Linda, California. For days afterward, Jan told visitors, "Hans says I can get well."

At 2:00 p.m., I planted another kiss on Jan's lips and left his bedside, spent. I was facing a *San Bernardino Sun* newspaper column deadline, so I retreated to the quiet privacy of our minivan to write. Here is what poured out of my heart:

When the "Good Life" Turns Bad
I'm writing this from our Ford Aerostar van in the parking lot of Memorial Hospital in Chattanooga on my little 540c PowerBook. Tears flow freely—and I stop every few minutes to wipe them away and blow

my nose. One can't cry well in the ICU waiting room surrounded by a blaring TV, anxious families, and the jangle of the phone.

Jan, my husband, suffered a massive stroke last night—February 8th. Fifty-nine. That's too young to lose the life you've always known. I started to say "the good life," but down deep in my aching heart, I'm hoping "the *good* life" is not lost, but yet to come. Different, perhaps, but good just the same. I need that hope right now—and so does he.

There is nothing I can do at the moment. He is sleeping in ICU—well-wired with monitors, oxygen, and catheter. Although I held his limp hand for an hour past the 12:30—1:00 visiting-hour schedule, the doors won't open again until 5:30.

Don't judge me for taking time out during a crisis like this to write. A bucket can only hold so many tears—and writing for me is therapeutic. In doing so I pleasure myself.

What do you do when "the good life" turns bad? Some of you reading this may be living in limbo like me: waiting for news of the condition of a child, spouse, or parent in some emergency room or ICU. Times like this are never anticipated, but statistics should tell us that sooner or later any one of us might be victim. Accident, disease, and disability are no respecters of persons. Have you considered what you need when life suddenly takes a drastic turn for the worse?

Family is important. Hold on to yours. Jan's and my parents are gone and our children scattered, but adopted family stood by me in the emergency room last night—and finally took me home about 1:30 a.m. And our closest child geographically, Kari, and her husband, Jeff, are on their way from Michigan. Our daughter, Kim, and her husband, Ed, and our son, Kevin, are monitoring the situation by phone, ready to come if needed.

Encouragement is second. The doctors shake their heads and talk about total disability or the fact that two-thirds of dense stroke patients either never improve or get worse. I may *need* the facts—but I *want* hope. Tell me about the one-third who made incredible gains, who exercised their brains in such a way that new pathways grew, who discovered new ways of doing old tasks. Tell me about the incredible power of our bodies to compensate, repair, and rebuild.

Third: Let me have some *time alone* to cry. I need to get in touch with my feelings. I need to mourn the loss. Chest-breaking sobs don't come easily in public.

Finally, *exercise* also helps. After the 8:30 visit this morning, I put on my Rebok shoes and walked around the hospital parking lot. With the sun shining in my face, I looked up to the blue of the sky and breathed in fresh air and was happy for a moment. I reached down and picked up a dime on the pavement. Good luck?

I don't know what the prognosis is yet. The doctors say "not good." But having Jan is good. He can talk. That's good. And his left arm and leg move. That's good too. And his kiss is strong. I can make this "the good life." I can savor the moments we have together.

I just hope your family doesn't wait for bad times—to savor the good.

Hope: A Welcome Companion

What is hope?

Imagine that you're struggling to keep your head above water in the tossing waves. Hope is the life preserver someone tosses to you with a strong rope attached that can pull you to safety. You're not in the lifeboat yet. But you're holding onto something that instantly changes your perception of what's happening to you. Moments before, you saw yourself being sucked down into the water, you saw yourself gasping for air, you saw yourself dying. You had no hope.

Now, with the life preserver, your situation has not changed significantly. You are still in the turbulent water, you are still gasping for air, but instead of seeing yourself dying, you see yourself being saved. And that makes all the difference.

With hope, you can live through terrible times without panic and fear.

With hope, you can fight on.

With hope, you have energy to overcome.

With hope, you see possibilities instead of impossibilities.

With hope, your circumstances no longer seem so bad.

With hope, you discover options you never knew existed.

With hope, you discover gifts and talents you never knew you had.

With hope, you shed discouragement and despair that pull you down.

With hope, you hold on to the positive expectation that everything is going to be OK. You don't know how, you don't know when, you don't know what's going to change. But hope gives you the confidence to live above it all, to view life from a God perspective, and to be content to follow in the Holy Spirit's wake—wherever that may lead.

The person who has lost hope in the future is doomed. George Kuzma, Jan's physician brother, observed this with one of his patients. He writes,

I once had a fiercely independent patient who had been ill for many years with adult onset diabetes and heart disease. She finally ended up in the hospital where it became apparent that the only way to save her life was to amputate her infected leg.

I presented her with the options: The first was that she could go on the way she was, and end up living in a nursing home where someone could take care of the progressive gangrene that would eventually take her life.

The second choice was to amputate her leg before it got to that point, which would mean that she could live a satisfactory life.

Her response was an emphatic, "No. I will not have it amputated, and I won't live in a nursing home!"

I tried to reason with her but she just turned her face to the wall. Reluctantly, I left. I was shocked to learn that a few hours later she had died. There was no acute reason for her immediate demise. She was in poor health, yes, but I had expected her to live from 6 weeks to 2 years.

I'm convinced she willed herself to die. How incredibly powerful are the thoughts of a person!

And then I discovered something Ellen White wrote on the power of the will. "By the exercise of the will power in placing themselves in right relation to life, patients can do much to co-operate with the physician's efforts for their recovery. There are thousands who can recover health if they will. The Lord does not want them to be sick. He desires them to be well and happy, and they should make up their minds to be well" (From: *Energized!* Compiled by Jan W. Kuzma, Kay Kuzma, and DeWitt Williams, Hagerstown, Md.: Review and Herald Publishing Association, 1997, 347).

Hope is what makes the difference! There is a very close connection between a person's state of mind and the immune system of the body. When hope and courage are lost, the result can be deadly. The will to live keeps the immune system alive; when it's gone, the forces of disease and depression have free reign, and death by natural causes or suicide is often the result. That's why there is an increase of death, especially suicide, around the holiday time. The person who is suffering keeps a glimmer of hope alive thinking things will be better by Thanksgiving or

Christmas. When it doesn't happen, and with only the long, lonely winter season ahead, many give up.

Hope is the substance a person must have to get through discouraging times. Without it, the will to live dissolves in the pain and uncertainty of the present. But hope, like happiness, is not something you grab for. For in grabbing for it, like a butterfly, it flits away. Hope is not an end in itself. It's the byproduct of finding meaning in the life you have been asked to live.

But what meaning could there be in suffering? Dr. Victor E. Frankl, who lived through the horrors of the concentration camps in World War II, gives some interesting insights in his book *Man's Search for Meaning*[1] about the meaning of suffering. When he was asked to make a presentation to his fellow sufferers in the last dreadful days before liberation, he began with the hypothesis that "our situation was not the most terrible we could think of." Here are the points he made to instill hope within the hopeless. Although the circumstances of our suffering are different, the same points apply.

1. *Very few of their losses were irreplaceable*. Most could be restored or achieved again, such as health, family, happiness, professional abilities, fortune, position in society.

2. Although their chance of survival seemed small (perhaps 1 in 20), *there was always the possibility that a great opportunity would come their way* quite suddenly. For example, they might be attached to a special group with good working conditions.

3. *What they had experienced, no power on earth could take from them*. He encouraged the prisoners with these words, "Not only our experiences, but all we have done, whatever great thoughts we may have had, and all we have suffered,

all this is not lost, though it is past; we have brought it into being. Having been is also a kind of being, and perhaps the surest kind."[2]

It can be reassuring to know that our suffering is not lost to the universe. The psalmist says, "You number my wanderings; Put my tears into Your bottle; Are they not in Your book?" (Ps. 56:8, NKJV).

4. *Human life always has a meaning*, and this includes suffering and dying, privation and death. Regardless of circumstances, life must be lived with dignity and meaning. When God looks down on them will He find them suffering proudly, not miserably, but knowing how to die? Even the sacrifice they were forced to make could have meaning if they chose to see that by their suffering, another was suffering less. Or perhaps by their courage, others would be blessed.

5. *Life is still expecting something out of you*. To give up and die would mean that someone in the future would suffer because they weren't there; the word of kindness would not be said, a friend would not be helped, the book would not be written, the piece of art would not be created. You can never be too sick, too disabled, or too old that God does not need you and what you have to offer.

Many are angry at God because they think He allows bad things to happen to, in some way, work out His master plan for the universe, perfect our characters, teach us important lessons, or punish us for our mistakes. But God doesn't make planes crash or boats sink, He doesn't cause children to be born with AIDS, or sentence thousands to die from starvation. All these things can be outcomes of troubles and trials, but it's not the reason for them.

The basic truth is, bad things happen to us because we are

living in Satan's territory. And the consequence of sin is death.

Jesus said it so well when He explained, "The thief does not come except to steal, and to kill, and to destroy. I have come that they may have life, and that they may have it more abundantly" (John 10:10, NKJV). Satan is the thief. Bad things happen because it's his agenda to steal, kill, and do everything possible to destroy our hope in Jesus, who promises to not only give us life but to give it to us "more abundantly"!

Here's how the apostle Peter puts it:

> Praise be to the God and Father of our Lord Jesus Christ! In his great mercy he has given us new birth into a *living hope* through the resurrection of Jesus Christ from the dead, and into an inheritance that can never perish, spoil or fade—kept in heaven for you, who through faith are shielded by God's power until the coming of the salvation that is ready to be revealed in the last time. In this you greatly rejoice, though now for a little while you may have had to suffer grief in all kinds of trials. These have come so that your faith—of greater worth than gold, which perishes even though refined by fire—may be proved genuine and may result in praise, glory and honor when Jesus Christ is revealed. Though you have not seen him, you love him; and even though you do not see him now, you believe in him and are filled with an inexpressible and glorious joy, for you are receiving the goal of your faith, the salvation of your souls (1 Pet. 1:3-9, NIV, emphasis supplied).

In other words: Our ultimate hope is the salvation that God has made possible through Christ's death and resurrection.

That's what gives us "inexpressible and glorious joy." Our trials just make our faith more genuine and pure, and our love for our Savior stronger.

With hope in God's plan for our salvation, one does not need to limit God's power in order to understand why bad things happen to good people, as Rabbi Harold Kushner does in his book, *When Bad Things Happen to Good People*. The critical element that Kushner left out of his argument was the great controversy between God and Satan that this world has been caught up in ever since Satan deceived Eve and Adam and won the right to have evil reign here for a time.

God has power to break through—that is the reason we experience the miracles we do. But God is also all-wisdom. He knows man and the universe must see the terrible consequences of sin. Evil must become so offensive and abhorrent to the watching universe that once it is destroyed here, it will never have a chance of breaking out anywhere else. And although I believe God wants good things to happen to us, His law is one of liberty that won't allow Him to take the freedom of another—even one who is torturing and killing others, as Hitler did.

Why does God choose to work a miracle for some and not others? God does not ask that we understand His ways, only that we love Him enough to trust Him and that we hold on to the hope that one day it will all be over. God's plan of restoring the earth to Himself, its rightful owner, is in the process of being executed according to His almighty power and His perfect timetable.

Why do bad things happen to good people? Because Satan reigns on this earth. Our only weapon of defense is HOPE. We can—in spite of what happens to us—live above it, hoping for the best, expecting God's blessings to break through, and celebrating the miracles, whether it be the saving of life or possessions or the miracle of being able to declare as Job did, "Though He slay me, yet will I trust Him" (Job 13:15, NKJV).

The author of Hebrews put it this way, "This certain *hope* of being saved is a strong and trustworthy anchor for our souls, connecting us with God himself" (Heb. 6: 19, TLB).

In my own search for answers to get through the unexpected challenge of Jan's stroke, I rediscovered 1 Corinthians 13:13, "And now abide faith, hope, love, these three; but the greatest of these is love" (NKJV).

I knew faith was important—it could move mountains—and I needed one moved. I was praying for the mountain of paralysis and brain damage to be removed from the man who meant everything to me. But I had no doubt, just as the apostle said, that love is the most important of the three. I felt creative energy and warmth when Jan looked into my eyes, when I snuggled next to him—or when I just sat there beside his bed watching the steady rise and fall of his chest as he slept. Together we could overcome whatever disability we faced. Together we could make it through anything. Love made it all worthwhile, regardless of how long and rough the road ahead might be.

But before the stroke, hope was an unknown to me—merely wishful thinking or an optimistic attitude. Now I began to see HOPE as the link between faith and love. Was it just chance that the apostle said Faith, *Hope*, and Love, and not Faith, *Love*, and Hope? Or Hope, *Faith*, and Love?

Hope, I discovered, is the positive expectation that keeps faith alive. It's what sees beyond the pain of loss to the gaining of deeper relationships. Hope is what makes one look to the stars above instead of the mud below and wish and dream and envision something better. It's what makes life worth living—and worth fighting for.

So it was, on that Friday after Jan's stroke, that I discovered through the encouraging words of a friend the incredible power of hope. Within moments, hope turned my blackest thoughts into technicolor possibilities. There was no significant outward evidence that Jan would get well. There was no official medical record that charted a trend toward wholeness. There was just the encouraging words of a friend.

Since that time I've thought about the power of those words. Hans could have been wrong. Jan could have been among the two-thirds of stroke victims who either stay the same or get worse. But even if that were true, hope would have made the journey easier. Hope would have cushioned the rough places I had yet to travel over. Hope would have soothed my shattered nerves and restored my sagging spirit with the courage I needed to meet whatever challenges I might yet have to face.

What a welcome companion hope was in my time of trouble!

But more than that, if Jan were to have the psychological and physical energy necessary to live a meaningful life and if possible, to recover, he had to have hope as well. He had to believe that regardless of how bad things were, there was something to live for. He had to believe that in the game of life, no matter how many times you're hit with crushing circumstances beyond your control or how many strikes the devil may have against you, with God you never strike out.

Months later when Jan and I reviewed our thoughts and

feelings during those critical first few days after the stroke, the analogy of a baseball game came up. Jan was born in Poland and grew up in Germany where he was a soccer champ among the kids in the displaced person's camp. So, it wasn't until he came to the United States when he was fifteen that he was introduced to the great American pastime—baseball. Here's one of his first memories after coming to this country—and I think it's an important one to hold on to for anyone facing an uncertain future.

I remember the first time I played baseball. I was attending summer camp at Camp AuSable near Grayling, Michigan. I was sixteen—that critical age when you try very hard to never get into a position where you could make a fool out of yourself, especially if any girls were watching.

I was up to bat. The last thing I wanted anyone to know was that I had never played baseball before. I had watched others play the game and knew how to stand and swing. So when the umpire called, "Batter UP!" I marched confidently to the plate, bent over slightly, tapped the plate, took a couple sample swings, flexed my arms, and looked into the eye of the pitcher. I was ready.

When the ball came over the plate I swung and hit the ball so hard that I cracked the bat. I hit the next one the same way; and the next. That's why a few innings later when the ball came toward me and I swung and missed, I wasn't prepared for the feeling of failure I experienced. When the umpire called, "Strike One!" I thought I would die.

After playing the game so successfully, I couldn't believe I had missed the ball. My confidence was now shaken; my cocky attitude was gone and my arms trembled a little as I waited for the next pitch. I was self-conscious now, for I knew everyone was looking at me. I felt like quitting.

I can't remember if I hit the next ball or not. I just remember the feeling I had when "Strike One" was called. I had let my team down. I chided myself, "What's wrong with you that you couldn't hit the dumb ball?" I felt like giving up.

Sooner or later there comes a time in almost everyone's life when the unexpected happens. When during your game of life you swing at the ball and miss, and someone yells, "Strike One!" Or maybe for you, it's "Strike Two," or even, "Strike Three!" The question is, will you keep playing the game with an "I Can" spirit and hopefully hit a homer? Or, with one or more strikes against you, will you give up and quit?

Jan had a major strike against him. Before, he was a successful biostatistician, researcher, teacher, administrator, the author of a popular textbook, and a statistical consultant for various projects. He was active in our church as a Sabbath School superintendent and teacher, a member of the school board, and was a respected thought leader on various committees.

He was also a doer. He was proud of his athletic prowess, whether it was on the tennis court, the volleyball court, or in the swimming pool. He was gifted mechanically and could fix or put together anything. Plus, he had a keen understanding of financial matters and had the ability to make wise financial decisions, which allowed me to donate much of my time to my Family Matters ministry, even though his salary as a professor at Loma Linda University was moderate.

In 1991 when we moved to Cleveland, Tennessee, Jan began Sentinel Research Services, a ministry to spread the health message through radio, consultation, and writing. Now he had the freedom to do everything he'd ever wanted to do in life. Then only five years later, everything changed when he had a stroke and the umpire of fate yelled "Strike One."

At first Jan's reaction was to deny this was happening to him. He just couldn't bring himself to believe that he'd had a stroke, and he told me so repeatedly. "Then why are you in ICU?" I'd asked.

That confused him. His only response was, "You think I had a stroke." Or if someone else asked him why he was in the hospital, he would say, "My wife says I had a stroke." But the idea of his believing he had a stroke was just about as absurd as his believing in Santa Claus.

Nothing could have been more shocking than Jan W. Kuzma having a stroke. He had none of the classic risk factors: He was in superb health, slender, and had normal blood pressure, and the last time he had his cholesterol level checked, it was 128. His veins were clean as a whistle. He had never smoked. He exercised daily. He ate a low-fat, mostly vegan diet. He lived a very low-stress flexible life in the country. No one told him what to do or when, and he made his own project deadlines. Plus, he was only fifty-nine. But it happened. He was stricken with the unthinkable. And the damage was severe.

Later, we learned that the number one risk factor for stroke for people Jan's age is now considered atrial-fibrillation—or irregular heartbeat. Five years earlier, when the atrial septile defect in his heart was repaired and he was given Coumidin, he either didn't believe what he heard or no one impressed upon him the fact that if he did not monitor his Coumidin levels regularly, he was significantly at risk for stroke. Now he was a victim of the very thing he was so sure he was preventing with his healthy lifestyle. The devastation of a stroke! His almost fatal mistake? He thought he would feel better on less medication, and by the time he consulted a physician, it was too late.

Now in retrospect, I wonder if his cutting back on the Coumidin for a few days didn't just hasten the inevitable. He was on such a minimal dosage—merely 2 mg per day, that he might have been flirting with the danger of stroke for a number of years, and sooner or later it probably would have happened! Maybe this was just a wake-up call to what could have been much worse. His doctor-prescribed therapeutic level of Coumidin is now 4.5 mg!

At first I was tempted to think, "What if he had monitored his Coumidin levels regularly?" But majoring in "What ifs?" only produces despair and guilt. What we needed to do now was move on with hope, making the best of whatever function Jan still had left, and to keep reminding ourselves when we were tempted to doubt what might happen to us in the future, that *"one strike doesn't mean you're out"*!

Yes, hope was a very welcome companion to both of us as we faced the challenging weeks and months ahead.

---

1. Victor E. Frankl, *Man's Search for Meaning* (New York: Pocket Books, 1963), 131.
2. Ibid.

CHAPTER
Three

I Call It a Miracle

While I keenly perceived and processed every movement Jan made—or didn't make, every one of his confused statements, and every physician's comment, trying to squeeze out every drop of hope I could, Jan, for the first couple days, was oblivious to the whole situation. He slept most of the time, and other than knowing something was wrong or he wouldn't have been in the hospital, he was in denial. I knew he disliked hospitals. Later he admitted thinking that if he could only get someone to unplug all the tubes and wires, he would have walked out. I'm just glad he didn't unhook himself and try!

Jan was sleeping Friday afternoon when Dr. Elden Chalmers, a pastor and clinical psychologist—and very special friend—came into his ICU room to pray for him. He laid hands on him and pled for his healing. Elden later told me that while he was praying he felt God's presence and was reassured that his prayer was in the process of being answered.

If I could pinpoint a beginning of the miracle Jan was about to experience, I believe it started that Friday afternoon. His left arm grew progressively stronger, and he was experiencing more movement with his left leg.

By the time our daughter, Kari, and her husband arrived about 10:30 that evening, he had experienced significant improvement in his ability to move. Kari gave him a quick evaluation based on her expertise as a physical therapist and with joy and excitement in her voice exclaimed, "Daddy, you can make it. You can move every muscle you need for recovery."

Then she immediately began to tell him what to do. "Daddy, take advantage of every possible movement you can make. Start with your face. Wrinkle it up, relax it, make a funny face. Then move your neck and shoulders. Make your left hand into a fist, squeeze, then relax. Wiggle your toes." But he was too tired to do anything after she left, and he slept until awakened by a nurse to check his vital signs then slept again.

By Sabbath morning Jan's situation had stabilized, and he was taken off the ICU monitoring equipment. Later that morning he was wheeled in for another CAT scan and then returned to room 164, and from that moment on until he left the hospital that next Thursday, I never left his side, except for a brief walk each day around the hospital grounds.

One never knows when he or she marries how one's spouse will react to tragedy. "In sickness and in health" is merely an expected cliché rattled off before guests, for at that peak moment of health and happiness no one expects anything except health and happiness "ever after." If one could see the future, one might not celebrate with such abandon, because life is uncertain. Bad things do happen to good people. None of us is immune to the strikes the devil would throw our way.

When Jan and I were married thirty-some years ago, neither of us had any idea Jan had a heart condition that would result in a significant part of his right brain being destroyed by a stroke. The bonds of marriage either break or strengthen at times like this. Ours strengthened. Jan knew he needed my smile, my encouragement, my help, and my enthusiasm for life to help him overcome whatever disability would be his. I needed his love, his tenderness, and his companionship. He felt sorry he couldn't do more to help me. I felt gratitude that he was alive. Over and over I said, "It's not function that matters, it's companionship." And we had that.

Plus, we had prayer coverage! By Sabbath, word came from around the world that family, friends, and strangers were praying for Jan's healing. At 3:00 Sabbath afternoon, nine pastors and elders assembled to anoint Jan with oil, as it says to do in James 5:14, 15 (NKJV), "Is anyone among you sick? Let him call for the elders of the church, and let them pray over him, anointing him with oil in the name of the Lord. And the prayer of faith will save the sick, and the Lord will raise him up."

What a comfort it was to me to put my complete trust in God that He could raise Jan up! God made Jan. He knew exactly what brain cells were damaged, and He could create new ones and restore Jan to his former state of health, if it was for Jan's ultimate good. Neither of us have any doubt about God's power. Knowing the elders had followed biblical instruction, anointing him with oil and laying hands upon him, made Jan feel especially close to God. These were the men he sat with on the church board. These were his friends. These were his spiritual mentors, his comforters, and his encouragers.

BLESSINGS AT MIDNIGHT

At the close of the service, Blondel took some pictures and Jan shook hands with each—using his left hand to show off the strength of his grip. Everyone said he looked good. Yet when we look back at those pictures, I realize how sick he really looked—very sick. But by Saturday night he was feeling better, and Kari was making him use his left hand to feed himself grapes. At first he picked them up using his four fingers against his palm. He was surprised that his hand had such a hard time finding his mouth. But by Sunday morning he had mastered his pincher grasp, using his index finger and thumb, and he could hit his mouth on the first try.

I stayed with Jan that night, and it's a good thing I did, because he was determined to get up to use the bathroom and take a shower. In the dim night light he could see the partially open bathroom door. In spite of the IV, the oxygen, and the catheter, he thought he could get up and walk to it. Sleeping on the cot beside him, I woke up several times to find his feet hanging over the side of the bed. When I asked, "Honey, what are you doing?" he said he was getting up. I tried to talk some sense into him, helped him scoot back up into bed, and covered him up again. But all he could think of is how good it would feel to feel the warm splash of a shower on his back, and he'd try once again to scoot out of bed.

I became concerned. What if I would sleep so soundly that I wouldn't wake up the next time he tried to get up, and he'd fall on the floor? What could I do to keep him in bed or make sure I'd wake up to stop him if he tried to get up?

Suddenly it came to me. His hospital bed looked big enough for two. I jumped off my cot, pushed aside the tubes, and crawled in beside him, putting my arm across his chest, so if he tried to move, he would wake me. Then I prayed, "Lord, please don't let the nurse catch me in bed with my husband!" It felt good to once again snuggle together, and we both slept soundly for the next few hours—only to be awakened by the nurse coming in to take Jan's vital signs. I couldn't believe she had caught me in bed with Jan, and I exclaimed, "I hope it's not against hospital policy to sleep with your husband!" She smiled and replied, "I wish more husbands and wives would sleep together. I think it's good for the patient to feel this closeness with their spouse. There's probably no other time in their lives when it's needed more!"

Well, that did it. Every night after that I'd wait until the new night shift nurse had done her rounds and then I'd get into bed with Jan and cuddle up. We'd pray together. And in the middle of the night when he couldn't sleep, I'd read to him. Dianne and Gary, my sister and brother-in-law, gave him Max Lucado's book *The Applause of Heaven* when they visited on Sabbath afternoon. So during the long hours of the night when Jan couldn't sleep, I would read to him—or he'd try reading to me by moving his finger along each line of words to keep his place. Every chapter seemed to be speaking specifically to us. By the time we left the hospital on Thursday, we were close to the end.

But I'm getting ahead of the story.

Sunday, Jan was able to bring his hands together as if to clap, instead of missing them in midair. And if he concentrated hard enough, he could get his left hand to touch his nose. With Kari's coaching, Charlene's encouragement, and the nursing staff's approval, Jan stood for the first time and shuffled a few steps to a chair and sat down. Supplemental oxygen was removed, which meant one less tube to worry about. And Kari made him eat his meals all by himself.

Jan was voraciously hungry each time food appeared, but eating wasn't as easy as one might think. Although he was still able to swallow, it wasn't quite the same as before the stroke. He stuffed in the food faster than he could swallow it, and I had to laugh at him when his cheeks looked like a chipmunk. He had no feeling on the left side of his face, and he couldn't tell that his left cheek was full of food. Many times throughout a meal, Kari would remind her dad to swallow what he had in his left cheek before taking another bite.

The stroke must have wiped out Jan's inhibitory response too. For over three decades I had lived with an incredibly disciplined man, extremely careful about what he ate and when, and now he'd eat anything—and everything! He couldn't seem to stop.

Monday, hospital physical therapy was begun and continued each morning and afternoon after that. Kari worked her dad hard in between, and his progress was phenomenal. That first day he had difficulty balancing, but he walked around his bed with a walker. The hand-to-mouth action on his left side was much improved, and his voice had more inflection and feeling in it and sounded less like a robot.

Kari and Jeff threw a going away party for Jan in the hospital that night, since *they* were "going away." They had to leave early the next morning and drive twelve hours back to their jobs in Michigan. They invited two friends, and we talked and laughed and enjoyed some great Chinese "takeout" food. Jan opened all the gifts Kari had gotten for him: Two sets of exercising outfits, five new colored T-shirts, and an exercise ball. She wanted him to feel good about the way he looked when he was able to leave Memorial hospital and be admitted to Siskin Hospital for physical rehabilitation.

I Call It a Miracle

In the midst of our party, Jan's neurologist, Dr. Farber, walked into the room. She was somewhat startled at the merriment and the empty bed. She came over to him sitting in the chair and asked how he was doing. She watched him eat, felt the strength of his grip, and then held her hand out in front of his left knee and asked him to try and kick her hand. He did. She looked surprised and said, "There aren't many patients who kick their neurologist!"

Since she hadn't seen him since Friday (it was her weekend off), she was obviously shocked, and pleased, at his progress. She then drew a picture of his brain on a napkin and indicated the spot where the clot hit and the large area where devastation was expected. "It must be luck," she said. "For some reason, the clot must have broken up and the damage is less than we expected."

Earlier that day Jan's cardiologist expressed his amazement at Jan's incredible recovery. And Dr. Don Mills, the radiologist (who had been one of Jan's students at Loma Linda University), after reviewing Jan's two CAT scans, put it this way, "The human brain has incredible potential, but this was certainly an act of God."

We called it a miracle!

Tuesday the intravenous medications were discontinued, and Jan was approved for discharge as soon as a bed was available at Siskin Rehabilitation Hospital, in Chattanooga. We grew increasingly impatient as we waited through Wednesday and still no bed was available. I got Jan dressed in his new jogging outfit, and I wheeled him all over the hospital in a wheelchair. Jan said the best part was getting outside, breathing the cold, crisp air, and seeing the sunshine. He was ready to begin living once again!

Finally, by Thursday Jan had improved so much that there was a question about whether or not he needed hospitalization at Siskin. By now all he wanted to do was to go home, and both of us were praying he could be accepted on an outpatient basis. Just one thing stood in the way: an evaluation from the hospital's physical therapist.

And then the most incredible thing happened. A cute, spunky physical therapist walked into the room and in a delightful accent introduced herself as "Agnes," saying she had the authority to determine whether Jan would need to be admitted to Siskin as a hospital patient or as an outpatient. I thought she must be Swedish or Norwegian and made some comment. "No," she said with twinkling eyes, "I'm Polish."

That did it. All Jan's anxiety vanished about whether or not he would be able to pass her evaluation. Jan immediately greeted her in Polish. She responded, and they conversed for a few minutes in their native tongue. She had only been in the United States a few years and intensely missed her homeland. With tears of joy welling up in her eyes, she said, "Your Polish is music to my ears."

Agnes Majewski ran him through all the paces: evaluating his balance, his strength, his shuffling walk with the walker, and his ability to get up from his bed and move to the commode—giving him all his instructions in Polish and he answering her in the same. Finally, she pronounced her verdict. "You pass," she said. "You did very well. *Bardzo dobrze*."

It took three trips to the car to carry all the gifts, fruit baskets, flowers, and plants Jan had been given during his week's stay in the hospital. Charlene wheeled him out and helped him into our green van. Then I got into the driver's seat and headed home to begin a new chapter of our lives.

I Call It a Miracle

On Friday, just one week after I was overcome with grief upon learning from the physicians about Jan's extensive disabilities, I noted on my computer: "Steady improvement with growing expectation for major recovery after intensive rehabilitation."

For my *San Bernardino Sun* column I wrote:

Miracles come in all shapes and sizes. Unfortunately, not every family experiences a miracle of healing as dramatic as Jan's. But every family, regardless of belief system can experience the miracle of a quiet spirit in spite of troubled times; hope when things seem hopeless; joy in the midst of sorrow, and a smile mixed with painful tears. These are remarkable events that cause one to marvel because they contradict the expected.

Too often family relationships, like life events, fall into predictable cause-and-effect patterns. He did this, so I'll do this. The miracle happens when the painfully predictable pattern is broken. Helping, instead of hurting the other. Instead of criticizing, encouraging. Instead of spiteful words, loving ones. And that miracle can start with you.

If you don't like what is happening "naturally" in your family, maybe it's time for a change. I believe in miracles. Won't you join me?

If Jan had been writing the column, his closing challenge would have been, "*I am a miracle!* You can be one too!"

CHAPTER Four

It Couldn't Happen to Me

When bad things happen, it's easy to say, "It couldn't happen to me." Bad things happen to others, but I'm strong, I'm healthy, I'm young, I'm a Christian—or for whatever reason, it couldn't happen to me! Perhaps it's wishful thinking, but we never think that fate will call a strike against us. Because we live in a world of sin, however, the chances are high that bad things will happen to you. And when it does, how will you react? Will you have the internal hope it takes and the external support and encouragement of others to find your way through the pain and heartache and emerge a better person?

In the early months after the stroke, if you had seen Jan, it would be easy for you to think, "Oh, Jan's the fellow who had a stroke." But that's not who Jan is—or what he wants to be known for. The stroke was merely the last paragraph in a long and far-from-finished book—and hopefully that paragraph will be a fleeting one!

A person should never be known for their disability but for their gifts; not for their handicaps but for their contributions; not for their productivity, or lack of it, but for the quality of their relationships.

For sixty years the hero in my story was Jan W. Kuzma, beloved son of William and Elizabeth Kuzma, admired brother of two older sisters, Donna and Christine, and a younger brother, George. He married the most wonderful girl in the world, or at least in Colorado (so he says) and became the father of Kim, Kari, and Kevin. He may have had a stroke, but he is still all of the above, and he always will be, regardless of whatever he may be forced to endure in the future.

Relationships, however, are only one way to describe a person. Another is by career: biostatistician, researcher, teacher, administrator, writer. Jan has been all of these—but that is not *him*. For career is only a flag along the road of life that designates a certain stage. It is whimsical: changing with education, interest, accident, or by a notice of termination.

Beyond relationships and career, we become who we are because of the life-changing events that come our way and the choices we make at these significant change points in our lives that ultimately form our character.

Nothing in Jan's life, other than the stroke, did more to chart the course he chose to take through life than the events that he experienced in his mid-teens. Not until you understand Jan from the perspective of who he was and who he determined to become will you realize why it was so hard for him to believe that he could have been the victim of a stroke.

Jan celebrated his fifteenth birthday somewhere in the middle of the Atlantic on the *General Harry S. Taylor*, a former military transport ship. It was his rite of passage. The year was 1951. He was leaving his war-torn childhood behind in the displaced person's camp in Wentdorf, Germany.

Gone were the reckless days of playing soccer until late into the night in spite of his parents' wishes; gone were the days of sloughing through school by the seat of his pants—getting spanked by his teacher for not knowing his lessons, being tattled on by his sister, Christine, and spanked again at home. Gone were the lazy days of pulling pranks and creating mischief, which happens spontaneously when there are no meaningful jobs to keep a boy's brain and brawn usefully occupied, and no purpose in life.

Now at fifteen, Jan was on his way, with his family, to the land of opportunity—the United States of America. For over six years his father had talked of nothing else except going to America: the land of milk and honey. For six disappointing years they had been hoping that the United States would grant them permission to enter her pearly gates. Now his father's dream was becoming reality. The ship, filled with European refugees, docked first in Caracas, Venezuela, and many disembarked. But the Kuzma family held papers for a better place. They were bound for the United States.

If there was ever a time to leave behind Jan's reputation for irresponsibility, it was then. Jan doesn't remember sitting on the deck of the ship, looking out over those endless waves and actually saying, "This is my chance to start a new life. I can make something of myself." But within him there was a growing feeling that he could amount to something. Maybe it's called maturity. Whatever, by the time the boat docked early that May 5 morning in New Orleans, Jan had determined that there was no obstacle so big that God and he couldn't conquer it. There was no job so skilled that he couldn't learn it; no task so tough that he couldn't do it; no field of study so difficult that he couldn't master it.

So armed with an English vocabulary that consisted of little more than "Please," "Thank you," and "Good morning," Jan walked down the gangplank with his first objective clearly in mind: to find, among that milling crowd of thousands, Mr. and Mrs. Ralph Jensen, their sponsors. He had no idea what they looked like. He had never seen their picture. He had no verbal description. Jan walked around for a while and then spotted a rather roly-poly couple dressed modestly in farming attire standing somewhat to themselves. He immediately went up to them and asked, "Mr. and Mrs. Jensen?"

Shock registered on their faces as they nodded their heads "Yes." Jan pointed to himself and said "Jan Kuzma" then motioned for them to follow him as he led them to where the rest of his family was waiting.

Something happened that day that changed the course of Jan's life. He became, in that one simple act of finding the Jensens on that New Orleans' shipping dock, the recognized leader of his family. His father was still the patriarchal head of the family; there was no doubt about that. But his family saw in him the street savvy that they desperately needed in order to get information and to make decisions in this new and very foreign land. That day they transferred their trust to Jan; a responsibility that he feels even to this day.

The Kuzmas were a city family, used to paved streets, the rush of commerce, and thousands of doors for Jan's father to knock on to introduce people to Bible truths by selling religious books and magazines. The little farm community of Elgin, Texas, in 1951 was a far cry from their comfort zone.

They had enjoyed beautiful hardwood furniture, delicate linens, and fine clothing when they lived in Poland, all of which they lost in pursuing their dream to come to this land of freedom and promise—a land "flowing with milk and honey."

Needless to say, after riding in the back of a truck over four hundred hot, dusty miles, the family was somewhat shocked when they were led to an old two-story farmhouse without indoor plumbing in the middle of a snake-infested cornfield and told this was their new home. They thankfully bathed in the creek (which they learned later was inhabited by water moccasins) and were thankful to have beds to sleep in.

They had nothing but their clothes and a few necessities—some dishes and linens—that they brought over with them in a trunk. Everything else was provided for them by the Jensens and generous church members. They had furnished the little farmhouse, provided shelves of home-canned goods and vegetarian meat substitutes, and made patchwork quilts on which was embroidered all the church members' names. The church had been anticipating their arrival and were happy they were finally there. But, for the Kuzma's, it was not "home."

The heat that summer was oppressive. They were now farm workers, and it was cotton-growing time. With temperatures soaring above 100, hoeing cotton all day in the burning sun for thirty cents an hour, was more than Jan's father could take. Plus, he missed being able to communicate with others in his native tongue. So he left that September to join Polish-speaking friends in Detroit. He found a job cleaning office buildings until he could learn enough English to once again do the work he felt called of God to do: spread the gospel by selling religious books and magazines as a literature evangelist. Shortly afterward, Jan's sisters followed their dad, leaving their mother, George, and Jan behind to fulfill the year's contract with the Jensens.

It was a good year for Jan. Everything he did, he did well, and his confidence grew. The first day picking cotton, the other workers laughed at him because his unskilled hands were so clumsy. But they weren't laughing at the end of the day when his load weighed in at seventy pounds, topping theirs.

Mr. Jensen asked Jan to do a number of jobs he had never done before, and he always came through with flying colors. Like the time Mr. Jensen asked Jan to take a load of cotton into town with the tractor. He didn't think to ask if Jan knew how to drive a tractor. He didn't. The scariest part, Jan says, was trying to get the load through the narrow entrance between the awning poles and the building. But somehow he made it, and Mr. Jensen was always quick to praise him.

For the first time in many years Jan found himself getting attention for positive achievement, rather than for his athletic ability or for his mischievousness. He was always figuring out a better way to do things, and Mr. Jensen liked that. One day Mr. Jensen was trying to catch a cow with big horns. He held the bag of sweet feed out, but when she'd put her head in and he tried to put the rope around her, she would spook. Jan watched for a few minutes and then asked, "Mr. Jensen. Let me try." Mr. Jensen handed him the feed bag and rope and stepped back. Jan tied the rope around the neck of the feed bag and held it out to the cow. As soon as her head was inside, he pulled up on the rope and caught her on the first try. Needless to say Mr. Jensen was impressed. "Jan," he said, "You and I will go into business together someday!"

But of all the lessons Jan learned out there on the farm, the most important to him personally was the lesson about the value of education. Jan really didn't want to spend the rest of his life picking cotton for thirty cents an hour. And the only ticket off the farm was an education.

In September when school opened, Jan began his daily walk of a mile or so to the main road where the school bus picked him up and took him to the high school in Elgin. In Europe, he never did very well in school, mainly because he was too busy having fun and playing ball to study. Now he found himself in an intimidating situation—taking classes in a foreign language. Jan studied hard and was shocked at the end of that first semester when he compared his grade card to those of his friends to discover he had made better grades in English grammar than they had. And he didn't speak the language—at least not that well!

That discovery turned his life around. He thought, *If I can do that well in a subject I know so little about, then what would happen if I knew the language—and studied hard?* The result was top scores throughout his academic career.

That next year when Jan, his mother, and brother joined the rest of the family in Detroit, Jan attended Wilbur Wright High School, a technical school that would allow him to get on-the-job training while taking high school classes. The school alternated one month of school and one month of working—for which he was paid. Jan graduated valedictorian of his class.

But to accomplish this meant that Jan had to make good use of his time. He became a very disciplined person. He put himself on a schedule and was even teased for his tenacity. On his seventeenth birthday, his sisters and friends threw a surprise birthday party for him, but since it wasn't on his schedule, he wouldn't come downstairs to enjoy the fun. To placate his sisters, Jan finally put in an appearance, but it was just to say Hello, then he went back up to study.

It Couldn't Happen to Me

It was also at this time that Jan became very interested in health. He knew if he felt good and could avoid sickness, he would be able to get better grades and accomplish more in life. He still remembered waiting in the long lines in the displaced person's camp for the health checks. Because of his family's deprivation during the war and the contagious diseases they had contracted, it took over six years before they could meet the health qualifications for U.S. entrance, and now Jan determined to do whatever was necessary to protect his health for the future.

Jan started reading the *Life and Health* magazines his father was selling. Every new health fact or lifestyle practice he learned about, he adopted. He gave up sweets, started exercising each morning and walking each night, and he made sure he got his sleep. Jan's mother had a fit when he became a vegetarian and wouldn't eat her good chicken soup. His refusal was a slap in her face. But he wouldn't compromise!

In college Jan's interest in health continued, so much so that he considered becoming a physician, even though he knew he grew faint at the sight of blood. Because of his spiritual leaning, many thought he should go into the ministry. But his natural talents kept pulling back into mathematics.

Jan prayed a lot during his senior year, asking God to lead him to the career most suited for him. But it wasn't until his professor Dr. Harold Jones showed him a letter from Dr. Frank Lemon, from The College of Medical Evangelists (soon to become Loma Linda University), that Jan found his calling. The letter said simply: "The College of Medical Evangelists (Loma Linda University) is going to be emphasizing more research in the future and we will be needing a biostatistician. At this time I do not know of any Seventh-day Adventist trained in this field. Therefore, I am interested in finding someone who is willing to become trained in biostatistics."

At the time Jan had no idea what a biostatistician was. When he learned that biostatistics was basically math applied to medicine; in other words, his area of giftedness combined with his area of greatest interest, he was excited.

It was during his master's degree work in the School of Public Health at Columbia, and then at the University of Michigan where he got his doctorate, that Jan became involved with research on lifestyle practices. Everything he learned he incorporated into his own life. Jan was deeply spiritual and believed what it said in 1 Corinthians 3:16 about the body being the temple of God. He wanted to present his body as a living and fit sacrifice for God's work. He wanted to spend his life researching the factors that helped one to live longer and live healthier. Jan felt to do so would bring glory to the Creator. That was his mission.

And that's basically what Jan did; first at UCLA and then for twenty-seven years at Loma Linda University as the chairman of the Department of Biostatistics in the School of Public Health. As he and Dr. Frank Lemon began to follow up some initial data that Dr. Lemon and Dr. Richard Walden had collected on a large group of Seventh-day Adventists, they found a six-year life expectancy advantage for those living the "Adventist lifestyle."

Immediately, Jan knew they were standing on a pot of "research" gold. This unique group of people who didn't smoke or drink and were either vegetarians or clean-meat eaters (according to Lev. 11) had something going for them that needed to be shared with the world. But who would listen, unless they had the scientific evidence necessary to "prove" what they already believed was the "Adventist Advantage"?

That's one of the reasons Jan's college buddy, Roland Phillips, after he finished medicine and his doctoral training as an epidemiologist, came back to Loma Linda University to work with Jan. They submitted many grant proposals together and received millions of dollars in funding. But the study that has had the greatest impact on our knowledge about lifestyle practices, health, and longevity was funded by the National Cancer Institute and later became known as "The Adventist Health Study." Today, Dr. Gary Fraser continues to direct this research, with new and exciting facts about health being published yearly.

Jan wanted the world to know that if people lived by the health principles God gave to His messenger, Ellen White, over a hundred years ago, they could live longer and healthier. In fact, using twenty-two years of follow-up data from that initial mortality study, they found that Adventists who participated in the study had death rates that were only 55 percent of the death rates of the general California population, giving a thirty-five-year-old Adventist male nine more years of life on the average. A later follow-up showed that vegetarians who watched what they ate, exercised and kept other health habits, lived thirteen years longer! Jan wanted the world to know that following what Adventists call the "eight natural laws of health" will make a difference: "Pure air, sunlight, abstemiousness, rest, exercise, proper diet, the use of water, and trust in divine power" (Ellen G. White, *The Ministry of Healing* [Nampa, Idaho: Pacific Press®, 1905], 127).

That's why, when he left Loma Linda University, he began writing a book called the *Live-Longer Lifestyle*. And that's why he started a daily syndicated radio program called "Got a Minute for Your Health?" heard on hundreds of stations around the world. The program was first hosted by Dr. David Grellmann and later by Dr. Elmar Sakala.

You might say Jan has a passion for health. It's not just head knowledge or a career for him. Health *is* his life. He has tried to incorporate everything he has had the privilege of learning into his own lifestyle. And that's why it was inconceivable to Jan—and everyone who knew him—that he could be the victim of a stroke!

But one strike doesn't mean you're out. And Jan's not going to quit now.

Jan's message to others is: Even though you may have one strike against you, don't quit! God can use you in an incredible way. What you are called to do may be difficult, and it may be different than what you originally thought. You may need to learn new skills or relearn skills, as Jan is doing, but you can do whatever God wants you to do.

As the year 1996 dawned, Jan thought because of his healthy lifestyle that he was invincible. If you had asked him about the possibility of a stroke, he would have said, "It will never happen to me! I will never have a stroke!"

He's been humbled now. It did happen to him!

Jan has never lamented, "Why me?" putting God on trial. Such questions only invite doubt, anger, and guilt. But we believe there is a reason behind whatever happens to us, even though we don't understand now. Perhaps Jan's stroke may be the avenue God chose to teach us another lesson we needed to learn to smooth out some rough edges of our characters.

Jan's prayer is, "Lord, do whatever You want to do to make me into the person You want me to be, to do the work You want me to do." That should be the prayer of all of us!

One Day at a Time

When major devastation hits, when you find yourself suffering from one of the big three—heart disease, cancer, or stroke—it's easy to get discouraged.

Or your "thorn in the flesh" might be a condition such as childhood diabetes, emphysema, epilepsy, or multiple sclerosis that is wreaking havoc with your life, and there is little medical science can do but ease your pain, mask the symptoms, and provide emergency care if needed. If that's your condition, you may be tempted to feel that life has cheated you.

Or it may have chronic pain—backache, migraine, or arthritis that keeps you from living the kind of life you'd like to live. Or your strike may be a relationship problem that can be as devastating as a physical malady; or perhaps you've lived to a ripe old age and your family feels you can no longer take care of yourself!

Since Jan's stroke we've discovered that there are

a lot of people who are suffering in this world, a lot of people who are far worse off than our situation. Scores of people who can't enjoy the sunset because their eyes can't see, can't relax to the melodic strains of a symphony because their ears can't hear, or can't even pleasure themselves by scratching where it itches because their arms or legs can't move.

I was shocked, when Jan shuffled into Siskin Hospital three weeks after his stroke, to see the condition of others who had suffered the same fate as he had. He was, indeed, one of the lucky ones. He was not bound to a chair. He had control of most of his body. He was just a little weak and a little uncoordinated, but he could move.

I saw one man struggling to talk, and as I listened it was almost impossible to make sense out of his uttering. I thought, *but for the grace of God, Jan could have been that man*.

I saw a middle-aged woman, not old at all, pushed in a wheelchair by her husband. I saw her fumble with her seemingly useless hands as she attempted the tasks she was asked to do, and in her frustration she ended up crying uncontrollably, and they had to send for a psychiatrist to quiet her. My heart ached with hers. But for the grace of God, Jan could have been that person—or it could have been me!

A number of patients couldn't eat by themselves, Jan shoveled in his food with ease—the result of three weeks of practice. But some we met had suffered such extensive damage that I knew they might never be able to eat like Jan. But for the grace of God, Jan could have been one of them.

And by far, most were alone in the hospital. When we asked where their families were, we were told they were "dropped off" and no one ever watched what they did in therapy. We were surprised. I never left Jan's side while he was in rehab.

I knew exactly the paces the physical therapist, occupational therapist, and speech therapist were putting him through. I had them copy instructions for me so we could do the same exercises at home. I felt sorry for those who didn't have that kind of support. But for the grace of God, either one of us could have been one of those who were fighting alone to regain function, rather than with the support and encouragement of a loving spouse.

When you are among those who are able; those who are pronounced "healthy" by whatever measuring rods medical science may use, it's easy to think, *It could never happen to me*. But I've learned that nothing in this world is forever. Bad things do happen to good people. Illness and accident does strike healthy people; and bouts of discouragement can even at times get the best of positive people. But you can cope if you'll just take one day at a time.

Since Jan's stroke, I've had a lot of time to think about life and what's really meaningful, and one of the things I've considered was the writings of King Solomon, who had the best of the best; who had wisdom and riches and everything one's heart could desire. Remember what he said about it all in the first chapter of Ecclesiastes? "*All is vanity*."

In the next few chapters, Solomon basically says there is a time for everything, but *nothing under the sun is forever*. You work hard and what do you get for it? Nothing, because regardless of what you do, you end up dying.

- That's why you should be happy with the things you do and what you have, rather than killing yourself trying to be like someone else or trying to accumulate more (Eccl. 3:22–4:8).
- That's why you should seek to have a friend or two;

59

because a companion will help you when you're down, keep you warm when you're cold, and protect you when you're in danger. In other words, a companion can make life worth living (Eccl. 4:9-12).

- That's why it's more important to be willing to learn, even though you might be poor, than to be a king who is set in his ways and won't listen to advice (Eccl. 4:13-16). Be flexible. So what if bad things happen to you? If you're willing to grow from the experience, it can't be all bad!

- That's why above all else you should seek to have a good relationship with God, because whatever God does, *it shall be forever* (Eccl. 3:14-15). People I know who have strikes against them have a deepened desire for heaven where all things are made new, where they will be given vibrant re-created bodies, and will enjoy eternity—forever and ever *pain-and-disability free*!

King Solomon summarizes his philosophizing with these words, "Here is what I have seen: It is good and fitting for one to eat and drink, and to enjoy the good of all his labor in which he toils under the sun all the days of his life which God gives him; for it is his heritage. . . . This is the gift of God. For he will not dwell unduly on the days of his life, because God keeps him busy with the joy of his heart" (Eccl. 5:18-20, NKJV). *The Living Bible* puts it this way, "To enjoy your work and to accept your lot in life; that is indeed a gift from God. The person who does that will not need to look back with sorrow on his past, for God gives him joy." That's good advice. And what a promise . . . *God gives you joy*!

Don't put off living today, thinking that someday in the future when your ship comes in, when the mortgage is paid off, when the kids are grown, when you retire, or when you feel better you will really begin living. Today is all any one of us has been given. We don't know what tomorrow holds. Today is the day to lift up your heart in praise and gratitude to God for that which you *do* have, rather than wasting precious time dwelling on that which you don't have. "This is the day the Lord has made, let us rejoice and be glad in it" (Ps. 118:24, NIV)!

That's why I'm so glad Jan and I never put off doing the things we really wanted to do. We never said, "Let's do it sometime in the future." We have no regrets. There is not one thing we can think of that we didn't do previous to Jan's stroke that we now wish we had done. We have lived every day to the fullest. Jan's stroke hasn't changed that.

Of course, there are still things we'd like to do, such as take a trip to the Holy Land or travel to Africa to see the herds of wild animals. But just because Jan's had a stroke doesn't mean we can't do these things. Just because Jan's had a stroke, we're not going to put our lives on hold. We want to continue living life to the max. Jan may not accomplish as much as he once did, but he can still experience the same joy—or even more—for each day that the Lord grants him. Regardless of how many strikes are against him—he's not out yet!

We have worked hard all our lives; but we have played hard too. There's not a time I can remember that we weren't planning some special trip with our family. Whether it was to Norway for our kids to sail on the *Anna Rogde*—the oldest sailing vessel in the world—or to Jan's homeland to visit General Wojciech Jaruzelski, the president of Poland, or to the island of Eleuthera to snorkel, sunbathe, and surf.

I once asked Kevin, our youngest, if he had any regrets about growing up with a working mother who wasn't there to greet him after school with homemade cookies and milk. "Of course not," said Kevin. "Who else gets to go to Hawaii for spring break?" And that's, indeed, what we've done. We have taken advantage of the times Jan has been invited to give presentations at conferences in various parts of the world or taken advantage of times when I have been asked to speak, and if possible, we've taken our children along. It's so important for them to experience the benefits of having working parents instead of bemoaning the disadvantages.

Although the children are older now and have lives of their own, we have continued this policy. It was our frequent flyer miles that brought all our family together, including Tristan, our three-week-old grandson, for two wonderful weeks in Kauai during Christmas vacation, just a month prior to Jan's stroke. We'll always be glad we did it, because life is different for Jan now. He's just not as active, as outspoken, and as authoritative as he used to be. And maybe that's good! But vacations now, because he's different, will reflect that fact.

We have continued to live each day to the fullest, trying not to let the stroke keep us from doing the things we love to do. Months before the stroke we had planned to take a trip to California on February 20. Kevin reminded his dad of this when he first called him after the stroke, "Dad, are you still coming out to see me?" Without thinking clearly about the seriousness of his situation, which included not yet being mobile, he answered, "Of course," and they continued to talk about the things they would do when they were together. After they hung up, I gently said to Jan, "Honey, we won't be able to take that trip. We'll do it when you're stronger."

I didn't say more. With Jan not thinking very clearly, and certainly not able to take care of himself, he knew he needed to submit to my better judgment. But he never gave up the dream. When he'd bring it up, I'd kiss him and say, "We'll go when you're stronger."

Jan wasn't surprised on Monday morning, the nineteenth (eleven days after the stroke), when I woke and snuggled up next to him and said, "Sweetheart, you're doing so well, and Siskins still hasn't been able to schedule you as an outpatient, would you still like to take that trip to California?"

"Of course," he answered. He was looking forward to seeing Kevin, who was attending La Sierra University, in Riverside, and his sister, Christine, who lives there. We also had other relatives in the area: my sister, Joanie, and brother, Rich, and their families. Plus, we had planned a week's vacation at Laguna Beach, the spot that held so many good family memories.

So I began to make preparations. A phone call to the commuter flights we were on gained the information that if Jan could climb up the seven or eight steps into the commuter plane, there would be no problem. He could be wheeled to the foot of the steps and then helped to his seat. His wheelchair would be waiting for him when he descended the steps. Although he hadn't climbed stairs since the stroke, I thought Jan had the will to manage.

On the twentieth he was still sleeping most of the day, unable to control his bladder and bowel function, confused in much of his thinking, unable to plan and initiate what he needed to do, and was exhibiting major signs of attention deficit. For example, if the TV was on, he'd sit glued to it for hours on end, watching indiscriminately. He wouldn't even hear me talking to him.

He also had difficulty understanding time concepts. He

would wake up Monday morning and think it was Friday. He had no idea about the passage of time and could sit for hours in one place just looking at his feet or dozing off and on but not initiating the movement necessary to get himself into a more comfortable position.

He knew he was supposed to exercise, but he was unable to sustain the activity. He needed someone to tell him almost every move to make. So, on the day of our departure, our friend Betty Hoehn, my "adopted" mom, came over and helped Jan with his exercises while I packed. I never complained about all I had to do, but I did comment to Betty, "I now know how a single mother with a small child feels, trying to get ready to go somewhere!"

Jan knew it wasn't easy for me to do all these things, plus give him the care he required, when I had been used to sharing the preparation for travel with him. But we were in this together, and I never wanted my husband to feel he was a burden. He wasn't. Being with him was a delight—even if it took a lot more work!

We made it to the airport, got on the plane, and then Jan decided he needed to go to the bathroom. This was a problem, because although he could sit down by himself, initiating the movement necessary to get back up was something else. He sat there on the tiny potty much of the first leg of our flight, with me outside the door asking, "Do you need any help?" Finally, I said in a voice that he knew meant business, "Jan, open the door." He did, and I pulled him up onto his feet. I doubt if he could have done it on his own.

In the Minneapolis airport, we searched in vain for a unisexual restroom so I could go in and attend to him. Finding none, I contacted a male attendant, and he wheeled Jan into the handicapped stall. I stood outside pacing the floor for twenty minutes waiting for Jan and the attendant to come out. Finally, I called in. "We're going to miss our flight." The poor flustered attendant said, "He won't get up."

So, I yelled, "If there are any men in there, tell them this is an emergency. I'm coming in." I waited a minute and then dashed into the handicapped stall and helped Jan. A number of men looked at me rather strangely when they saw me exit the men's room!

Our son, Kevin, picked us up at the airport in Ontario, and when we pulled up in front of Jan's sister's house, I got the wheelchair ready for Jan, but instead, he said he was walking to the door, and with help, he did. We carried the wheelchair all over Southern California and never once used it then carried it all the way back to Tennessee!

One of the things Jan has had the most difficulty with since the stroke is figuring out how things work. One of the most confusing has been water faucets! In our shower in Tennessee, there is just one lever to regulate the temperature. At first, I had to really watch Jan to make sure the water was not too hot or too cold, or he'd either freeze or burn himself. After a few showers, he learned what to do, and even though his reaction time was slow, he could get the right temperature.

But during that first visit to his sister's house, he never learned how to regulate the two shower knobs. No matter how many times I showed him, "out for on, in for off, left for hot, right for cold," he never could figure it out. One time when I got busy and he got into the shower by himself, he nearly got scalded before he could get out. When I came in a few minutes later, the bathroom was steaming, and he was leaning against the wall outside the shower stall, shaking from fright. He knew he was getting burned in the shower but couldn't figure out what to do. Let me tell you, after being a person who could do anything and could figure out anything, it is scary when you can't even figure out something as simple as how to operate water faucets! My heart ached for Jan at that moment like at no other time after the stroke.

Well, as it worked out, we had a wonderful time in California. Just two weeks after the anointing service at Memorial Hospital, we took pictures of Jan walking on the beach at Emerald Bay. Who would have thought he would have such a remarkable recovery in that short time! We purchased a small motor home, and I drove back across country so we could stop by Colorado and visit our daughter, Kimberly, her husband, Ed, and their baby, Tristan. We left their place on Sunday afternoon, thinking we had plenty of time to drive the 1,400 miles to make our nine o'clock appointment at Siskins Rehabilitation Hospital in Chattanooga, Tennessee, on Tuesday morning.

But we had an electrical problem with the motor home, and the taillights kept shorting out, making it very dangerous to drive at night. I stopped numerous times to try to get it fixed, but no one could find the problem. Finally I grew desperate, thinking we would miss our first rehabilitation appointment, so I drove until 2:00 a.m. Tuesday morning with the hazard lights blinking. Then I pulled into a motel parking lot to sleep a couple hours, thinking I would wake up in time to make it to Chattanooga for Jan's appointment.

The next morning when I woke up and looked at the clock, I screamed. I had slept an hour later than I had planned. Of course, Jan had no idea what time it was—nor what day. He was merely along for the ride, so he wasn't concerned. But I was panicked—and drove like Jehu. We barely made it, pulling into the Siskins' parking lot at 9:02 a.m. with the wheelchair that Kevin and his cousin, Jeff, had tied on the top of the motor home.

After two weeks of practice, Jan was now walking fairly well. And that was a good thing. It took a lot of effort for me to climb on top of the motor home, tie a rope onto the chair, and let it down over the side all by myself. It's tough to do things alone, when you've always had someone else take that responsibility. But I learned I could do it, and I feel better about myself because of it.

I'm telling you all this to make the point: *If you really want to do something, you can do it*, but you've got to believe it's possible. If you say "It's impossible," you'll never put forth the energy and creativity necessary to figure out how the impossible can be possible. We once heard Leland Kaiser, a health administration consultant, say, "Every assumption can be proved false."

We have adopted that philosophy as our own. I could have assumed, "With Jan's condition, it's impossible to go to California," and we would have stayed home, and Jan would have missed all the positive stimulation of visiting his friends and relatives and seeing our children. But I didn't. We proved the assumption that "we couldn't go" false, and we went. And the memories will last a lifetime.

Misery is wholesale. Look around you, and you'll find people suffering. If you happen to be one of those whom society has pronounced "healthy" and you don't interface often with those who have suffered a strike or two, pay a visit to your local hospital, rest home, or rehabilitation center. It will be good for you. You'll appreciate more the health that you have. Nothing is forever. When you see someone worse off than you, remember . . . but for the grace of God, it could have been you.

During the last couple years, my friends and acquaintances have carried many burdens. Here's just a sampling:

- A wife has a rare type of skin cancer with no known effective treatment. Wait. Wonder. Worry.
- A young mother finds herself divorced. The father of her child is now remarried and has a new baby daughter. He shows no interest in his five-year-old, who thinks the world of her daddy. How does this mother explain that the child's father has rejected her? How does she cushion the disappointment when there is no Christmas or birthday gift? What does she say when her daughter asks why Daddy never comes to see her when he lives just a few miles away?
- Son died of AIDS.
- The scaffolding collapsed. A fall, and an active, vibrant 36-year-old husband and father of two school-age boys is confined for the rest of his life to a wheelchair, never again to move his extremities—a quadriplegic.
- A young wife with a darling curly headed three-year-old son left her husband. Four years of putting up with his alcohol and marijuana abuse, citations for "driving under the influence" and "in possession of . . ." was too much for her; four years of heartache hoping tomorrow would be different; hoping that her husband would give up the habit that is cruelly ruining their lives.
- Wife has Alzheimer's. A fiftieth wedding anniversary came and went—but no recognition. He has cared for her in this condition for the last four years, but as her condition deteriorates, he's facing the decision of placing his beloved sweetheart in a convalescent center. His heart is breaking.

68

One Day at a Time

I once heard a story about a man suffering with a heavy burden. Seeking relief, the man asked his guardian angel if he could but exchange his burden for another's. The wish was granted, and he was led into a room filled with other people's burdens. One by one each burden was examined and discarded. The man finally left with his own.

As tough as life is, most of us would not choose the lot of another. We must take comfort in the fact that we have not been given more than we are able to bear. Jan may have suffered a stroke, but as heavy as this burden is, we would not exchange it for the misery of any of our friends.

We've found that humor helps to get us through discouraging moments. Jan's sixtieth birthday came in April, just a few months after his stroke, and he was surprised when his brother, George, and his family gave him a Dr. Seuss book. He hadn't read one since our kids were small. With a sense of wonder, he opened *Did I Ever Tell You How Lucky You Are?* and began laughing. His favorite page shows an ominous forest with the branches of trees reaching after a pantless fellow who is running away. One branch has plucked off the poor guy's pants. Here are the accompanying words:

And suppose that you lived in that forest in France,
where the average young person just hasn't a chance
to escape from the perilous pants-eating-plants!
But your pants are safe! You're a fortunate guy.
And you ought to be shouting, "How lucky am I!"
(Dr. Seuss, *Did I Ever Tell You How Lucky You Are?*,
[New York: Random House, 1973], 39.)

Yes, even with a strike against him, Jan knows he's a

very lucky guy!

The secret to accepting your condition in life, whatever it may be, is to just take one day at a time. If we were to think of that every day for the next thirty or forty years, Jan would feel as washed out as he feels right now, limping through life, experiencing difficulty with simple body functions like bladder control or worrying that his heart could throw another clot, life would not be worth living. *But today is not that bad.* That's why Jesus said, "Therefore do not worry about tomorrow, for tomorrow will worry about its own things. Sufficient for the day is its own trouble" (Matt. 6:34, NKJV). The Living Bible puts it this way, "So don't be anxious about tomorrow. God will take care of your tomorrow too. Live one day at a time."

Regardless of the misery or pain that may be your lot, you, too, can make it through today. That's all that is asked of you. Circumstances change. Miracles happen. People grow. Wounds heal. Life goes on. Hold on to today. Meet the challenges you or your family face today and grow better, not bitter. Nothing is forever; and *anything can be borne, one day at a time*.

And in Dr. Seuss's words:

> That's why I say, "Duckie!
> Don't grumble! Don't stew!
> Some critters are much-much,
> oh, ever so much-much,
> so muchly much-much more unlucky than you!"
> (Dr. Seuss, *Did I Ever Tell You How Lucky You Are?*,
> [New York: Random House, 1973], 48.)

CHAPTER *Six*

The Incredible Power of Prayer

When bad things happen, I'm often reminded of a quotation I memorized years ago that goes like this: "We have nothing to fear for the future, except as we shall forget the way the Lord has led us and his teaching in our past history" (General Conference Daily Bulletin, "We Had a Hard Struggle," January 29, 1893).

There is tremendous hope that can be found within each person. There is no life so miserable, so painful, and so abused that you cannot see the hand of God at work in some way, sometime in your life, if you would just ask for spiritual insight.

What has God done for you in the past? When you were a child, could you see God in the embrace of a mother, father, or grandparent? Or perhaps God broke through to you in the smile of a friend? Perhaps you fell in love and felt within you the desire to give unselfishly to another. That's divine. Without God working in your life there would be no love. Just because you may have lost that love, just because suffering may have come your way, does not mean that God was absent then or is absent now.

It's like the story told about the footprints in the sand: At times in your life there are two sets—yours and God's. But when the suffering is the most intense, there's just one set because God is carrying you—even though you may not know it. When in your past can you imagine that God may have been carrying you? It's from those times that you can now draw on to find hope for the future.

After my mother's death from an automobile accident where I was the driver, a fellow sojourner sent me this poem by Janet Chester Bly. I found myself immediately identifying with it!

> I would rather clutch my invitation
> and wait my turn in party clothes;
> prim, proper, safe and clean.
> But a pulsing hand keeps driving me
> over peaks, ravines and spidered brambles
> So, I'll pant up to the pearled knocker
> tattered, breathless and full of tales.

The past shapes our future—either for good or bad—depending upon how we choose to allow it to affect us. We have that freedom. It's our responsibility to look back to the times when God was there and hold on to that. Our lives are a testimony. God has given each one of us a story from which we can draw strength. And in the sharing of our stories, others can find hope by the way God has led us in the past.

Which brings me to looking once again at what it was in my husband's life that gave him such a strong faith in God.

What made him a man of prayer? Why is it that even when struck with a massive stroke, his hope never wavered?

Jan's faith in a God who answers prayer is not a Pollyanna faith or merely wishful thinking. It's based on personal experiences from childhood where there was no doubt in his mind that God reached down and changed the course of history as a direct result of the prayers of his family.

His mother taught him to pray. It wasn't that she was more spiritual or a more deeply committed Christian than his father. It was just that she was around a whole lot more during his earliest years, while his father was out "doing the Lord's work" selling Protestant books, magazines, and Bibles in Catholic Poland.

That combination of a Protestant zealot, like William Kuzma, bicycling around Catholic Poland selling what the priests considered heretical material was like pouring gas on hot coals. There were bound to be explosions. That's why almost every time his father came home from one of his trips he brought with him incredible stories of answered prayer; how, in spite of persecution, his father was able to share Bible truth. So there was never a time Jan didn't believe in the mighty power of God.

The first time, however, Jan really remembers his folks pleading with the Lord was when he was eight years old and his father had just gotten word that the Nazi army was subscripting him into a forced labor camp. They had hoped the war would end before the inevitable happened—that their father would be taken. After all, Jan's father was almost fifty years old. But as the summer of 1944 approached, the Nazis were suffering great losses. They were desperate for manpower and were taking every able-bodied man, regardless of age. So the family pleaded for their father's safety. The Nazis hated the Polish, and the only thing that had previously saved Jan's Polish father was his mother's German background. In a labor camp he wouldn't have that protection; the Nazis treated animals better than the Poles.

Jan's father had to go; there was nothing the family could do about that. And after a few months they lost track of him, but it never entered Jan's mind to doubt whether or not God heard their prayers. They simply believed that God would take care of their father—as well as the rest of the family—and they never ceased praying.

The war ended, but the story of God's intervention in the Kuzma family did not. At last the family heard Father was alive in a German displaced person's camp, and he wanted his family to escape from Communist Poland and join him. Miracle after miracle followed this family from one crisis to another, each adding to Jan's shield of faith. So by the time Jan came to this country, God and he were on good speaking terms, and Jan trusted Him implicitly.

But it was during the summer between Jan's sophomore and junior college years that Jan literally prayed without ceasing. He never felt called to be a literature evangelist, selling religious books and magazines like his father did. But because of an interesting chain of events, he ended up doing that very thing.

With his experience working in various engineering plants, plus the engineering courses Jan had taken in high school and college, he thought it would be easy for him to get a full-time summer engineering job in the South Bend, Indiana, area where there were so many plants. He filled out twenty-six applications, but after receiving the same number of rejection notices, he began to wonder what was wrong.

Feeling defeated, he left college for his home in Detroit. On the way he remembered the chapel talk given by the literature evangelists who were recruiting students for summer jobs. They promised that with six or seven hours a day, students should be able to obtain a full scholarship for the following year's tuition. He needed work, so he called the literature evangelist office to inquire. Carl Hobson, a successful literature evangelist, came out, trained him, and a few days later sent Jan out by himself.

Jan was motivated, there was no doubt about that. He had to live up to his father's reputation as one of the most successful literature evangelists in Poland. His mother, who also had done this work, had an equally impressive record. The last thing Jan wanted to do was come home at night and face his folks, especially his mother who always asked, "How much did you sell?" and have to say "Nothing!"

Yet, that's exactly what happened the first day—and the second—and the third. Jan began to put in twelve- and thirteen-hour days, and he prayed harder and longer than he had ever prayed before in his life. He prayed without ceasing, and yet three weeks went by and still no sale. There had never been anything Jan couldn't do, and now it appeared he was a failure in the very work where his folks had incredible success. Mother even began to wonder aloud, "Jan, perhaps you're just not cut out to be a literature evangelist like your dad. Perhaps you're not made of the same stuff!" That hit hard.

Finally, just to make a sale Jan gave a large discount on a small children's picture Bible. He just couldn't face his mother one more night and tell her he hadn't sold anything.

You'd think he would have given up. But not Jan. As long as God and he were working together, he didn't consider himself a failure. He just prayed more and worked harder!

Shortly after that, Jan knocked on the door of a Nazarene preacher. He looked through the books and said "These are wonderful Christian books. I'd like each member of my church to have a set" and gave Jan a letter of introduction to his church members, along with the church directory. From then on there was no stopping the Lord and Jan. *They* made big sales of whole sets of books worth two hundred or three hundred dollars. By the time school started, *they* had sold over five thousand four hundred dollars worth of books, more than any other student literature evangelist in the Lake Union during the summer of 1957.

Jan had worked at many jobs, but never before had he felt he was truly doing the "Lord's work"—nor had he prayed so unceasingly. As a literature evangelist he prayed before, after, and with every contact he made. And God blessed. Because of his work hundreds of families now had good religious books in their homes to help them develop positive Christian values in themselves and their children.

This experience taught Jan something about God's ways. He believed that with his first prayer for success in placing Christian literature in the homes in Detroit, God was in the process of answering. But God's timetable was not Jan's. Jan wanted a sale immediately. God's answer was "wait."

One of my favorite texts explains why God sometimes says "wait" to a prayer that He is in the process of answering. It's Psalm 50:15. *The Living Bible* puts it this way: "I want you to trust me in your times of trouble, so I can rescue you, and you can give me glory."

If Jan had made a sale immediately, everyone would have praised Jan. Or they would have given the credit to natural ability, "After all, his folks have both been very successful literature evangelists. He's just a chip off the old block." And if Jan were an immediate success, he wouldn't have felt the urgent need to pray without ceasing. As it worked out, there is no doubt in his mind the reason for his ultimate success. God had heard his "time of trouble" prayers and answered, and there was nothing else Jan could do but give God the glory.

God is indeed able to do "exceedingly abundantly above all that we ask or think . . ." (Eph. 3:20, NKJV). This is a powerful promise to hold on to when you're in a dark valley of your life and desperately need hope!

During those tough teen years as an immigrant boy trying to make it in a strange country, Jan found his faith strengthened by reading the Bible and inspirational books. He read *The Desire of Ages,* about the life of Jesus; *Patriarchs and Prophets*, about such greats as Abraham, Jacob, and Moses; and *Prophets and Kings,* about Elijah, Elisha, and David and other Bible heroes. But of all the Bible greats, Daniel was his favorite. He found hope in patterning his life after Daniel's. Jan thought they had a lot in common. Daniel was forced from his home by a foreign invasion, just as Jan was. He found himself in a new country, just as Jan did. Daniel was interested in healthy living, just as Jan. Jan even copied Daniel's example of praying three times a day. And just as Daniel never compromised his principles, Jan determined to do the same.

Attending a public high school was not always easy for a Christian teenager. Jan's peers did many things he would not even consider. Some cheated to get better grades, while others experimented with harmful substances such as alcohol and smoking. These were not issues for Jan. Like Daniel, he had determined to stand true. And like Daniel, Jan felt God was continually rewarding his faithfulness with good health and a capable mind. Jan wasn't doing these things for a reward. He just wanted to live his life to the best of his ability, according to what he knew was right.

The closest Jan came to having a lions'-den experience was when he was working in the machine shop for the Dodge truck manufacturing plant and was faced with whether or not he would join the labor union. Jan had been an employee for several months and was making over six dollars an hour—very good pay for a seventeen-year-old who was not yet through high school. Jan knew it was expected that all employees would become dues-paying union members, but he kept delaying this decision because he felt Christians should not be members of organizations that used violence to force decisions. By joining he would become a so-called union puppet, doing whatever the union boss said, regardless of his own individual convictions. Jan believed he would be going against God to give up his right to determine what he should or should not do according to his conscience.

One day the supervisor, who respected Jan's work, spoke to him about joining the union. He said that the other guys had been talking about Jan, and two of the union members would be coming during the lunch hour to discuss the situation with him. The supervisor looked worried—and because of the stories that were circulated around the plant about what happened to employees who refused to cooperate with the union boss, Jan was scared.

The guys who talked to Jan were husky, rough-looking blue-collar workers, who made their position clear. Either he joined before tomorrow or they would send the Flying Squadron to see him. Jan asked if he could give the money for dues to another organization like the Red Cross, and they laughed.

After the workers left, Jan discussed his options with his supervisor. He was told that the last guy the Flying Squadron confronted had been badly beaten. Although that wasn't exactly the lions' den, it was close enough, and Jan really didn't like that option. He would not give up his principles, but unlike Daniel who had no other option, Jan did. That night when he left work, he never returned.

Finding another job where Jan wasn't going to be forced to join a labor union was not easy. He finally found work mixing cement for a small construction firm. The job was the hardest work he had ever done in his life—for a lot less pay. It consisted of carrying eighty-pound sacks of cement, ripping them open, mixing them with sand and gravel, and carrying the cement to the construction site. It was backbreaking work.

Jan needed the money, however. He knew he wanted to attend a Christian college and his folks weren't able to help him. Therefore, he endured the backbreaking work in order to pursue his dream. He was most grateful a year later when September came around and he had earned what he needed to travel about two hundred miles southwest to Berrien Springs, Michigan, to begin four wonderful years at Andrews University—then called Emmanuel Missionary College (E.M.C.).

Jan had worked hard academically and physically for four years to be able to go to a Christian college. Nothing could deter him, not even the army. When he turned eighteen on April 24, he registered with the local draft board as the law required. A few months later when he was packed and ready to leave for college, he got an unexpected response from them. The formal letter was short and to the point. He was being drafted into the army and was supposed to report for induction in a few days.

Jan was shocked. This was not part of his plans. He prayed for wisdom. The day he was supposed to be reporting for duty was the same day he was to be registering at E.M.C. He had no time to appeal. He had to make a decision. Jan chose college and wrote this short note to his draft board:

> "Dear Sirs: It was with surprise when I opened your letter requesting that I report for induction into the Armed Services. Unfortunately, I will not be able to be there because I have been preparing to attend Emmanuel Missionary College for the last four years. My bags are packed, and I'm ready to go. I would appreciate it if you would reconsider my case and allow me to get my college education, since I will be able to serve the U.S. Army better following my graduation. Yours truly, Jan W. Kuzma."

Jan realized his letter was fairly presumptuous. He knew the army was like the IRS; what they said was "law." But he did what he thought God wanted him to do; he enrolled at E.M.C. and prayed daily that God would intervene with the draft board. Two weeks later, their response was forwarded to him. "Dear Mr. Kuzma: The draft board reviewed your suggestion, and it is my pleasure to inform you that your request has been granted. Please continue with your college education and let us know of any change of address."

Once more Jan felt like Daniel. He had stood for what he felt God wanted him to do, and God worked things out. But what if God doesn't work things out for you? What if you pray and your hope for the future is dashed on the rocks? Or what if the pain doesn't go away? Or maybe your child doesn't come back to God?

God doesn't always break through and change the natural course of events. He didn't with Daniel. I have a feeling Daniel prayed he wouldn't be carried off to Babylon as a captive—but he was. Does that mean God is dead? No it doesn't. Perhaps it just means that God has something special for you to experience in the circumstances you are called to endure. Perhaps the miracle is not in the events themselves but how you are able to deal with the events.

God never refuses a prayer for courage, steadfastness, compassion, endurance, patience, and understanding. He never refuses to be with you wherever you're forced to go and whatever you're forced to suffer. Sometimes it helps to understand God's mysterious ways to review how He worked in the lives of Bible heroes.

Who is your Bible hero? You may have chosen Abraham, who left his home to follow God's calling, or Moses, who was probably one of the most able leaders and administrators who ever lived. Maybe you are praying for a double portion of God's spirit, like Elisha did, and would like to be used by God as that humble farmer turned prophet was. Then there is John the Baptist—the most outstanding evangelist who ever lived; or Lydia who was known for her humanitarian service to others. There are many to choose from. But if you would go through all the possible Bible heroes and rank them according to whom you would choose to be like, I have a feeling which one would probably be at the bottom of your list—Job.

As honorable as Job was, as faithful in spite of tragedy, pain, and the negative influence of friends and family, no one who is currently healthy and enjoying the good life would ever wish to be like Job.

When you're young and have the world at your command, it's easy to see yourself as a modern-day Daniel, as Jan did. But when bad things happen, the story of Job and how he handled loss, pain, and disability becomes much more intriguing. If you're needing an extra dose of hope, Job may be the hero you need to pattern your life after. Could it be that what you are experiencing has more significance than what you currently perceive?

Why was it that God opened the windows of heaven, so to speak, and allowed us, through the story of Job, to catch a glimpse of the heavenly conflict between good and evil? Could it be to give us an insight into what is going on behind the scenes in each one of our lives? Could it be to help us to be more understanding when bad things happen? Could it be a way of testing our faith?

I was first alerted to the parallel between Job's life and Jan's when I read the paraphrase of the second chapter of Job, substituting Jan's name and condition for Job's.

I could just imagine the scene where the administrative angels responsible for various inhabited worlds were attending God's heavenly executive committee to give a report. Satan comes representing the earth. When it's time for his report, he starts bragging about the fact that he has such control over his earthly subjects that no one is keeping God's law anymore; and even if they did, they certainly wouldn't do it because they loved and trusted God.

Then I can imagine the following conversation between God and Satan.

"Have you considered My servant Jan?" the Lord asks. "He is one of the finest men in all the earth—a good man who fears God and turns away from all evil. And he has kept his faith in me despite the fact that you persuaded me to let you harm him without any cause."

"Skin for skin?" Satan replies. "A man will give anything to save his life. Touch his body with sickness, and he will curse you to your face."

Confronted with this challenge before the whole universe and knowing the test would be good for Jan, God reluctantly replies: "Do with him as you please; only spare his life."

So Satan goes out from the presence of the Lord and strikes Jan Kuzma with a massive stroke. And in spite of the physical and mental devastation, this modern-day Job declares, "Though He slay me, yet will I trust Him" (Job 13:15).

And the story continues:

Then within minutes of the time this faithful man of God is struck, prayer chains ignite across the world as the people of the earth rise up with one great cry, beseeching God to heal His servant, Jan.

And that, indeed, is what happened in Jan's case. The gates of heaven were barraged by a massive force of praying family, friends, and strangers around the world. It was not until days and weeks later that I realized the magnitude of this praying force, as phone calls, letters, and e-mail messages started pouring in.

The ASI (Adventist-Laymen's Services and Industries—an organization we belong to) administrative board was at Pine

Springs Ranch in southern California when they got the word about Jan's stroke, and immediately business stopped and they were in prayer for Jan. The same thing happened at Andrews University, Jan's alma mater.

John Reinhold, the executive director of Christian Care Ministry, the organization we belong to where Christians share each other's medical needs, and his wife, Dona, were immediately on the phone to me, uplifting Jan in prayer, and assuring me that all Jan's medical needs would be taken care of. That in itself was an incredible answer to my prayers. I had heard horror stories of the hassles others had with their health insurance companies in getting the bills paid then sometimes learning that not all was covered.

But the Medi-Share plan was different. In addition, John and Dona informed me that Jan's name had been placed on their prayer alert list, and he would be uplifted around the clock as Christian Care Ministry members called the 1-800-PSALM33 number to learn who needed prayer.

The question is, how do prayers make a difference in the great controversy between good and evil that is being fought over our lives? Just this: You could argue that Satan won the earth "fair and square" as his territory and he and his evil angels have the right to reign here. After all, Adam and Eve sinned. But God has the power and the angels necessary to destroy these evil beings— if He would choose to do so. But force is not a part of God's government. Instead, I see God waiting and wanting to break through and help us, but at times holding back His attack unless we ask for help, and in a way give Him our permission (as Satan's subjects) to disregard Satan's jurisdiction.

When God hears our prayers and acts, and when something good happens which we would not expect in this world of sin, we call it a miracle. And that's what I believe happened in Jan's case.

I can imagine the good and bad angels struggling beside his bed: the good wanting to bring the blessing of healing; the bad trying to protect "their" territory. As the waves of prayer began to flood heaven, the good gained strength and began to over-power the evil. Finally, as the prayer power increased, Satan and all his evil angels had no recourse. They were powerless to stop God's blessing of healing from being poured out.

Why doesn't God, in every instance when there is heavy prayer coverage, break through into Satan's territory? I don't know. God's ways are not our ways. We are not called to understand God—only to love Him and trust Him. But some-day when God explains these events from His perspective for the ultimate good of His people, I'm sure I will agree with the way He called it.

That's really what faith is all about! Knowing without a doubt that God has the power to act, giving Him our unceasing prayer permission but letting Him call the plays, and saying, regard-less of the outcome, "all things work together for good."

I believe, when God's people pray, Satan is powerless.

Although the end of Jan's Job-like saga has not yet been written, I like what scripture records about Job. "So the Lord blessed Job at the end of his life more than at the beginning" (Job 42:12, TLB). I trust God that He is in the process of do-ing that for Jan. And I trust that regardless of what situation you find yourself in, He is doing that for you.

I believe that just like Job of old, there is a battle going on for each of us. Satan brings our names before God and says, "No wonder he or she follows You. Look at the way You have been blessing that person all their life."

Although God won't force Satan to stop tempting or harassing you, you can be assured that God is faithful and "will not allow you to be tempted beyond what you are able, but with the temptation will also make the way of escape, that you may be able to bear it" (1 Cor. 10:13, NKJV). That's good news, isn't it?

And to me, whatever affliction may come my way, whatever strikes may be called against me, it all seems worthwhile if God can use my case to show the universe that I will love and trust Him, regardless. Although there is suffering in this world because God may not interfere with the natural process of disease, alter the consequences of our own negligent actions, or even take away the freedom of choice from an abuser, that does not mean God isn't carrying you. What you can be assured of is that God will always answer your prayer for personal courage to deal with the suffering, joy in spite of pain, and hope when things look hopeless.

The question is, when a strike is called against you, will you stand firm?

God is wonderfully good. Crisis is never anticipated; pain is never planned. Yet tough times come to all. But through it all, God is there and His Word speaks to us words of comfort and encouragement if we will only take advantage of His gift. In this time of anguish and loss, Jan and I found hope in Lamentations 3:21-23:

"Yet there is one ray of hope; his compassion never ends. It is only the Lord's mercies that have kept us from complete destruction. Great is his faithfulness; his loving-kindness begins afresh each day. My soul claims the Lord as my inheritance; therefore I will hope in him. The Lord is wonderfully good to those who wait for him, to those who seek for him. It is good both to hope and wait quietly for the salvation of the Lord" (TLB).

CHAPTER Seven

All Things Work Together for Good

Why is it that some individuals seem to rise to the top when bad things happen to them, while others get buried with discouragement? Why is it that some who have a strike or two against them grab the opportunity and carry it to victory, while others bend to defeat?

It was quite uncharacteristic for Jan and me to be watching TV late at night, but the 1996 U.S. women's gymnastic team was in a neck-and-neck race with the Russian team for Olympic gold. Even if we had gone to bed, we wouldn't have been able to sleep not knowing the result.

Never before had the U.S. been so close to the gold. To win the team gymnastics gold medal would be a first in the 100 years of Olympian games. The U.S. team trailed by only a few tenths of a point. All the pressure of the last week of competition fell on seventeen-year-old Keri Strug, the last gymnast to vault. She had two tries to make it—her highest score would count. If the score were high enough, the U.S. would win the gold medal. If not, Russia would take away the coveted prize.

Keri's first attempt was a dismal failure. She didn't complete the final revolution and instead of landing on her feet, she fell backward on the mat. But the strike against her was worse than merely the psychological pain of failure in front of millions of onlookers. When she fell, she badly sprained her ankle. Close-ups caught the wince of pain on her face as she limped off the mat. She had one more try, but it was obvious to everyone watching that the U.S. was doomed. How could Keri compete with a sprained ankle? By default Russia would win.

But the competition was not yet over, and one strike didn't mean that Keri was out. Limping into position, Keri readied herself for what she knew she had to do. She had one more chance to win, and she was going to take it.

In disbelief, Jan and I watched as she sprinted down the mat, vaulted into the air, and executed a perfect landing on one foot! Then falling on the mat she gripped her ankle as sharp pains riveted through her body. But her courage, determination, and skill had secured the gold for the United States.

I wonder, if Keri didn't think she'd make it, would she have gone through the pain? If she didn't have the driving dream to hope for the gold, would she have tried that second vault?

I've thought a lot about what it takes in life to succeed when you have a strike or two against you, as Keri had. And this analogy came to mind. It is as if when a strike is called, the road before you forks. At that point you are presented with a choice. You have two possible paths you can take. One is the path labeled "All things work together for bad" and the other "All things work together for good." Everything after this point will be determined by the path you choose. Everything will be affected by your attitude.

The well-trod path is the first. It's the natural response. We live in a world of sin, so obviously bad things are going to happen. People who see the negative side of life live by the philosophy that "It can't get so bad but that it can't get worse." Or in the words of that old baseball song, "It's one, two, three strikes, you're out . . ." That's it. You're doomed to failure.

Those who take the road less traveled choose the opposite response to bad things. They declare, "All things work together for good," even though it may not look that way. In making this choice, they are immediately freed from debilitating worry and fret. They can rest in the Lord and find the peace He promises, even in the midst of the terrible battle between good and evil, health and sickness, or life and death.

Choosing to look at life positively is like knocking down the first domino in a line. When that goes, the rest follow. Without deliberate planning, positive thinkers begin to take responsibility for making sure that "good" does, indeed, come from the bad. Whatever strike is called against them, they stay in the game doing their best to hit the ball and hopefully make first base—if not a home run.

Keri took the road less traveled. She made "good" out of "bad" and won the gold. I prefer to live by the same philosophy. Jan and I have had many strikes against us in our lives, but we're not going to let them get us down. And we're certainly not going to let this stroke get the best of us either.

Jan's first big strike against him came when he was seventeen years of age. He had worked hard at the jobs he held during his sophomore and junior years of high school and had saved three thousand dollars. That was a lot of money for a teenager in 1954. Jan had come to the U.S. three years before with nothing but the clothes on his back, which he was quickly outgrowing, and now he had enough money to make some kind of an investment. But what? Jan decided that real estate would be a good way to have a steady income. For example, if he bought an apartment house, the rent would not only make the payments but would bring him additional income. So he began to search the classified section of the *Detroit News* for possibilities.

The ad said, "Income-producing property available," so Jan called. The agent showed him an apartment house that was for sale and gave him a song and dance about what an incredibly good buy it was, especially when you could get five hundred forty dollars of net income each month. Without consulting anyone to determine the truth of her statements, Jan determined it would be a good investment and gave her three thousand dollars as a down payment.

The nightmare started when he tried to collect the rent. That first month he was shocked to discover that even if everyone paid what was due, the amount was far short of what the agent had promised. In fact, it didn't even pay his bills. But the worst part was trying to get the rents paid. It was like trying to squeeze water out of a turnip. A white, foreign-born teenager must not have looked much like an owner of an apartment building in an all-black section of town. Regardless of what Jan did, most people just wouldn't pay him. They refused to open the door. Or they said, "Come back tomorrow." They treated him like scum. And one big, burly man even pulled a knife on him.

Jan's usually not a quitter. He attempted to collect rent money for three months and finally he couldn't take the cursing and abuse any longer. Without rent money, he didn't have the money to make payments, and seeing the handwriting on the wall, he went to talk to an attorney about his options. When it became clear there was no way for him to maintain payments for the property, Jan decided to give up his three thousand dollars down payment (the most money he had ever had in his life) and sign the property and his nightmare over to the lawyer.

Jan felt like a failure, but he didn't sit around and mope. Instead, he began to list the lessons he had learned.

Lesson 1: Real estate was still a good investment opportunity, but he would never again buy something without consulting a number of knowledgeable and experienced people.

Lesson 2: He also learned you can't believe everything the salesperson tells you. Do your homework thoroughly before making a commitment.

Lesson 3: Don't invest in something where you are dependent on the money of others for it to succeed. For example, he would never again get into a position where he had to collect rent from a hostile clientele.

Lesson 4: Avoid investing in property in poverty areas where the property value is going down; not up.

Lesson 5: Don't put all your eggs in one basket—diversification carries less risk.

I'm not sure these lessons were worth three thousand dollars. But Jan has made a number of successful real estate investments since that time, and following the lessons he learned as a seventeen-year-old, he has more than made up for that loss.

While Jan's first testing of the truth of Romans 8:28, "all things work together for good to those who love God," had to do with money, the second had to do with love.

When Jan was in high school he became intrigued by the expressive writing of a young woman columnist of a church paper and on impulse wrote to her. She responded, and thus began a writing relationship. Her words were beautifully chosen; her insight was impressive, and before Jan knew it he was in love with the person behind the pen, although he had never seen a picture of her or met her. When she wrote that she and her mother were coming to Detroit, they arranged a meeting. But when Jan met this girl, he was shocked. She was sickly and mentally slow, and he quickly realized that her mother had been doing the writing. As incredible as it seemed, this mother had the idea that they should immediately be married. But marriage was the farthest thing from Jan's mind. That experience made him shy away from any girl who looked the slightest bit interested.

When Jan went to college he wanted to be polite but quickly found that with even a little show of kindness or attention, the girls latched on to him like leeches. So after a few dates, he decided it wasn't worth it and vowed to never date another girl until he was ready to get married. Jan began his sophomore year with a no-date policy but quickly found it a rather lonely way to live. There were events on campus where it would have been nice to have a friend to accompany him. So he modified his policy and decided that if he could find a girl who was dating someone who was not on campus, she would not be interested in him and, therefore, she would be a safe person to take to various functions.

About this time Jan met someone whose boyfriend was

attending college elsewhere, so he asked her out, clearly explaining that if for any reason she and her boyfriend broke up, he could no longer go places with her. It was a convenient arrangement for both of them, and it continued into his junior year. Then partway through his junior year, she told him her boyfriend broke up with her. Jan reminded her of their agreement, and he stopped seeing her.

It was not until they didn't see each other, however, that Jan realized how much he had grown to depend on her presence. Like the famous line from the film *My Fair Lady*, "he had grown accustomed to her face." Both of them were miserable, and so Jan buried his policy of not dating someone "available." By his senior year they were going steady and not long after that he asked her to marry him.

This was not a hasty decision. Jan had prayed earnestly about whether or not this girl was to be his wife. At first Jan had some doubts, and then he did a foolish thing: He prayed that God would give him a sign. Then he opened his Bible and read something about "God blessed this house" and took that text as a sign from God that this was the right girl for him.

But when her old boyfriend returned, she became confused. She said she loved Jan, but she was torn between her two boyfriends. Their relationship began to rock with the whimsy of her emotions. When the old boyfriend was around, she broke up with Jan. Then when Jan ceased to write or call, she thought she couldn't live without him and said she would give up the old boyfriend. But throughout this time, Jan was really never concerned. He had his sign from God (so he thought), and he waited for her to make the "right" decision.

When her final decision was for the old boyfriend, Jan

couldn't believe it. How could that be? Had God let him down? Jan questioned, but he never gave up his trust in God. It took time for him to see how foolish he had been to let a Bible text make the decision about whom he should marry, when God had given him a perfectly good brain for those kinds of decisions. It was a valuable lesson for him.

Once again, "all things worked together for good . . ." for it was only a few months later that he noticed a girl singing next to the piano in the parlor of the girl's dorm at La Sierra College in Southern California. She had long blond hair, was dressed in a lovely gray suit, and her voice sounded to him like heavenly music (so he told me later). He stopped momentarily to watch her (for she looked very much like his old girlfriend), and his sister, Christine, noticed.

Christine, who was attending La Sierra, had arranged three blind dates for Jan on that weekend he was visiting her in California. He had no time to work in a fourth date, but he was strangely drawn to this girl.

"Do you want a date with her?" Christine asked.

Trying not to sound too interested, Jan replied, "Sure, but how are you going to get rid of one of the other ones?"

"I'll see what I can do," Christine replied.

What Christine didn't tell him is that she had already noticed the similarity between me and Jan's old girlfriend, and when one of the blind dates she had arranged weeks before had fallen through, Christine had invited me to be the substitute blind date for their Sunday outing.

"All things work together for good." And this substitute blind date certainly did. I might be biased, but I think we were much better suited for each other intellectually and psychologically than the old girlfriend. Our interests, our talents, and our dreams jived. I've told Jan many times throughout our thirty-some years of marriage, "I'm so glad I looked like the old girlfriend!"

The third testing of the truth of the text, "all things work together for good," had to do with Jan's career. For a man, career means everything. It defines who he is. He may be husband and father, but he's introduced as Dr. Jan W. Kuzma, chairman of the Department of Biostatistics at the School of Public Health, Loma Linda University, while his wife is often introduced as "Mrs. Kuzma," regardless of her career.

Jan had given twenty-seven years of his life to Loma Linda University. He had been especially chosen and trained for a position at Loma Linda and was one of the founders of the School of Public Health. Through the years, he had been responsible for numerous funded grants bringing in over two million dollars of research money into the university. Jan not only was the author of many published scientific articles, but he had also written a biostatistics textbook and was a popular teacher—if you can ever call a statistics teacher "popular!"

He had been active on the faculty senate and on various university committees, was the director of Research for the School of Public Health, and was a tenured full professor. His position was secure. By all academic standards, twenty-seven years after he began with Loma Linda University, Jan was at the height of his career.

Then in 1989, they closed the school, and Jan's job was terminated! No one could believe it! It was a known fact that finances were tight, but after all those years, this turn of events seemed impossible to our friends and colleagues. But there was no mistake.

Throughout the years, our children on occasion would say

to Jan, "Daddy, you are so smart, why don't you get a job were you can make more money?" His standard reply was, "God called me to Loma Linda University. My mission field is my students, and until the Lord calls me elsewhere, this is where I will be." You might say Jan was committed!

A few weeks after Jan's termination notice, the administrators who were responsible for closing the school (thinking they could reopen it under the umbrella of the School of Medicine with fewer faculty) found that if they went through with their closure plan, accreditation would be lost. That would mean financial suicide. What student is going to pay tuition for an unaccredited program? They had no choice, therefore, but to reopen the school.

Jan's job was reinstated. But he no longer had a feeling of commitment. After twenty-seven years, it was gone. So a few months later, the university allowed him to take the consulting work he had established, and he formed a nonprofit organization, Sentinel Research Services, which now produces a daily radio program called *Got a Minute for Your Health?* and allows him to do statistical consultation and write health books and articles.

Why was this so good? Just after this happened, my organization was asked to move to the Cleveland, Tennessee, area to develop Welcome Baby, a friendship evangelism program for families with newborns. If Jan had still been teaching at Loma Linda University, it would have been very difficult to make the decision to move to Tennessee. But as it turned out, he was self-employed and could take his work anywhere. Now Jan and I love the South. There isn't a morning when we get up that we don't express to each other how blessed we are to be in beautiful Tennessee. Neither of us has ever regretted the move.

But we have been doubly blessed. Now Jan is free to travel with me to my speaking appointments rather than being tied down to an eight-to-five (plus) job with all the personnel and administrative hassles. Working for himself, instead of another institution, until retirement age, has been like having ten extra years of his life handed to him. God is good.

And it was because Jan was terminated that I urged Jan to go see Dr. Raymond Herber for a complete physical examination while our health insurance, which he had never had reason to use, was still in effect. That exam led to the discovery of Jan's atrial septal heart defect. The timing was critical. The standard procedure was to have it repaired with open-heart surgery. When Jan said he didn't want surgery, Dr. Jutzy knew of a colleague, Dr. Charles Mullins, in Houston, who was doing an experimental procedure where they go in through the vein in the groin with a patch for the hole in the heart. The mechanical patch is all folded up as it goes up to the heart and then when it gets into position, like two umbrellas on both sides of the hole, they open it, pull it together, and the hole is patched.

Jan went to Texas Children's Hospital, since this was a procedure usually done on children, and avoided open-heart surgery. A year or so later, we heard the procedure was no longer being done because an FDA committee charged with the responsibility of maintaining a check on the effectiveness of new medical procedures was concerned about a technical difficulty.

If Jan's heart condition had not been discovered at that time, he might have had a heart attack and died. It could have been discovered too early, and no one would have had an alternative to open-heart surgery; or too late and the experimental procedure would have no longer been available. But no, the timing was perfect.

BLESSINGS AT MIDNIGHT

As we look back on this unfortunate chapter in our lives, we have to wonder. Many people have questioned why the administration of Loma Linda University did such a seemingly foolish thing as to close the school before finding out the ramifications to accreditation and then have to backpedal and quickly open it again. I don't. I know why! God allowed it in order to break Jan's commitment to the School of Public Health, so He could move us on to the new work He had for us to do.

Just because one is able to say "all things work together for good" doesn't mean that there isn't a good deal of pain attached to the unfortunate event. Eight years later when we were attending a marriage workshop, the couples were instructed to experience Romans 12:15 where it says, "Weep with those who weep," by asking their spouses to describe the saddest thing that ever happened to them in their lives. I was surprised after Jan having lived through the Nazi invasion of Poland and then escaping from Communist Poland that he said as tears started streaming down his cheeks, "The saddest thing that ever happened to me was being fired at Loma Linda!" We both wept.

It might be easier to believe "all things work together for good" in the areas of finances, marriage, or career, but what about when your health is destroyed? How can having a stroke be good? Every person who suffers a stroke has a different experience, but we've spent a great deal of time thinking about the stroke Jan had and how possibly this strike against him could be good. In Jan's own words, here are a few of the ways:

1. My greatest desire in life is to be ready for Christ's second coming. If this stroke can help smooth out the

rough edges of my character, it is little enough of a price to pay.

2. Legalism can't save you; only God can. Living a legalistically healthful lifestyle is not bulletproof protection against disease. Satan is the author of disease and death, and as long as we're living in his world bad things are going to happen to good people. This stroke has humbled me. I no longer think of myself as better than others because of my healthy lifestyle. Nor do I see myself as invincible. Only by the grace of God are any of us kept from the devil who is running around like "a roaring lion seeking whom he may devour." (See 1 Pet. 5:8.)

While legalism won't save you—since there are no 100 percent guarantees—I still believe you are far less likely to suffer disease if your immune system is healthy. I believe with all my heart in the following natural remedies: a good wholesome diet, rest, exercise, not drinking or smoking, pure water, fresh air, sunlight, and trust in God. And many have told me they feel it was my healthy lifestyle that has helped restore my lost functions so quickly.

3. I am much more sympathetic and understanding to those who have a strike or two against them.

4. This stroke may have served as a wake-up call. As massive as it was, it did not totally disable me or kill me. By taking care of myself now and monitoring my medication, I may have prevented an even bigger stroke.

5. My children now have a father who is a better listener, not so quick to give advice, and one who has

time for them and the grandchildren.

6. I have received hundreds of encouraging letters, e-mail messages, and phone calls, many from people I didn't know. I had no idea people cared about me so much that they would lift my name up in prayer. What a treasure friendship is!

7. Kay feels more competent to manage our affairs in case something worse happened to me.

8. I'm not so tied to deadlines as I was; projects mean less to me now than people do.

9. I've had a chance to do a lot of reflective meditation and praying. I'm stronger spiritually for having gone through this experience.

10. Although good things have happened to me, I never before felt I was a miracle. Now I know God has stepped into this world and touched me in an incredible way. I stand with a select few who can truly say, "God performed a miracle and healed me."

When it began to sink into my head that I had, indeed, had a stroke, Kay asked me what I believed were the extent of my disabilities. My response was, "It all depends on what God wants for me and my belief in what God can do for me." It never entered my mind to doubt.

God knows far better than I what I need for the building of my character. He also knows what bad things He can trust me with, that I will not be overcome, but that together with Him, can make something good out of it. I can, even when bad things come to me, thank God that He can trust me; that I will take the positive fork in the road and not let

Satan's darts of disability get the best of me.

When bad things happen, "all things will work together for good" if we believe it. But this is only true if we choose the right fork in the road—the positive one.

Romans 8:28 doesn't say that God is responsible for making sure that all things work together for good, while we sit back and mumble and moan over our unfortunate state of affairs. But it does say that "all things work together for good to them *that love God.*"

Loving God is the key. If you love God, you will believe His promises. You will spend time reading and memorizing encouraging Bible texts that you can repeat over and over until they become a part of you. You will pray that God will make you a better person because of what has happened to you, rather than a bitter one. And in doing so, you will set God's natural healing process into motion as energy-giving endorphins are released into your system.

I believe we as God's children have a responsibility to make sure "all things work together for good," and believing this becomes a self-fulfilling prophecy. When we choose the positive road, we'll find the good in the bad, we'll experience the truth in Solomon's words, "A merry heart does good like a medicine," and the whole world will be a better place because of it.

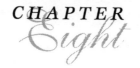
An Anchor in the Time of Storm

Since I was a little girl I can remember singing the old hymn . . .

> "Will your anchor hold in the storm of life,
> When the clouds unfold their wings of strife?
> When the strong tides lift, and the cables strain,
> Will your anchor drift, or firm remain?"
> (Seventh-day Adventist Hymnal, 534).

Of course, the song is about being anchored to Jesus our Savior—the Rock which cannot move—and the importance of being grounded in His love. Through the years I've discovered there is incredible truth to these words; that if I just hold fast to Jesus I can survive whatever crisis, pain, and loss Satan throws at me.

But there is another anchor that can help you get through the stormy times in your life. We rediscovered it after Jan's stroke. The anchor is *family*.

When the big storms in life have hit me, it's my family that is the anchor that helps me hold on to my faith and keeps me from being dashed on the rocks of discouragement. It's my family that lifts me up when I'm down. It's my family that helps me feel secure when it seems that my world is crashing down around me.

When I need heaven to reach down and hold me, Jesus does it through the hugs of my husband and my children. He does it through the phone calls from my brother and sisters, the letters and notes of encouragement from my extended family, the prayers of my church family, and the support and care of others who treat me as a sister.

When I asked Jan about whom he felt in his life had been an important anchor, he immediately replied,

My first anchor in life was my mother. I was only eight when our family was caught in Poland as the Russian and Polish troops forced the Nazis to retreat back through Poland. When I tell the story of my Polish father being taken by the Nazis to a forced labor camp, when I tell how my mother and we four children survived when we were forced to leave our home and how we finally escaped from Communist Poland, people always ask, "Weren't you afraid?"

When I was first asked the question, I was surprised. Fear? I had really never thought of it before. "No," I answered. "As long as Mother was with us, there was nothing to fear." I knew there wasn't a problem too big for her and God to solve. I had perfect confidence in her ability to protect us from the enemy.

I knew she and God were very close, so I had no reason to feel insecure.

When our world came crashing down on us, my mother, who had cunningly used her German background to gain favors from our Nazi captors during the four years of their occupation of Poland, was now finding the tables turned. When the Russian and Polish front recaptured Plotz, our beautiful city on the Rhine, no "friend" of the Germans would be safe from the pent-up fury of the Russian soldiers and the revengeful Polish people. Without our Polish father to protect us, there was no doubt that our lives were in danger. So we left everything behind, and in the gathering darkness of that frigid wintry night in January, we rushed to the train station, hoping that we could get out of town before the Russian and Polish troops marched in.

Was I scared as I clutched my baby brother's buggy as the cattle car lurched forward, away from impending danger? Not really. Excited, yes, and cold. But not scared. Mother was there.

I've found through the years that the biggest enemy a person can have is not financial disaster, displacement, or disease; it's loneliness. Hope is always alive when you have someone who loves you. But when you're alone, you're extremely vulnerable to thoughts of hopelessness and despair.

That's why divorce and death are so devastating to the survivors. That's why it's so important for a church family to adopt the singles and provide supporting security nets—social networks—that keep those who have no immediate family from crashing in the pit of discouragement.

I think that's why Jan rallied so quickly after his stroke. He was never alone. Except for that first day in ICU when visiting hours were restricted and he slept almost continually, I was always there; his anchor during the worst "storm" of his life.

Jan says my presence meant the most to him during the night hours. When he would wake in the middle of the night and sleep evaded him, time dragged. He said just listening to my deep breathing was comforting. He knew I was there if he needed me. He was not alone in his suffering.

Jan said he wasn't afraid of being alone. He could have made it through the nights by himself. Even though he often woke to consciousness with some confusion, when the confusion cleared, he knew there was a nurse somewhere down the hall who would talk to him through the wall speaker if he hit the emergency button—*if he could find it*—and help would eventually appear in person. But there is a difference to the psychological quality of the interaction between paid service and love service. Both may perform the same acts; both may have the same skills; but when it's family, the interconnections, the bond, the history we have shared makes the psychological quality of the interaction entirely different.

I understand now, as I never did before, why hospice is so important when life is ebbing away. To die among the familiar, with family, is to die on a much higher psychological plane than in the presence of machines, monitors, and technicians, regardless of how skilled they might be.

Family is the anchor in the time of storm; it is an important shelter from doubt, anxiety, and hopelessness. It is the life jacket that keeps us from drowning in loneliness.

I have always prided myself for being able to take care of my own needs. But being alone, even if one can cope, is certainly one of the lower levels of existence. God knew what He was saying with His pronouncement, "It is not good for man to be alone."

I don't believe any family who survives medical crises is ever the same again. No marriage stays static. Jan and I grew closer. Before, being capable, secure, and responsible individuals, we often traveled separately; I to my speaking appointments, Jan to his conventions and professional consultations. During our child-rearing years, since our children were our priority, we reasoned that it was best for one of us to be home with them most of the time.

We thrived on being confident and secure enough that we could exercise our freedom without threatening our relationship. Indeed, it grew. There is nothing like a few days of separation to make our hearts and bodies yearn for reunion. On each flight home, anticipation mounted; each embrace after a time apart was like celebrating a minihoneymoon. But things are different now. Medical crisis has brought with it a new level of interdependency. The "need" on Jan's part, the "want" on mine. And that feels good.

The incredible thing, as I canceled my appointments and took off that next year to devote my time to helping Jan get the therapy he needed to regain as much function as possible, is that the Lord took care of the Family Matters ministry. At the beginning of the year, the *Got a Minute for Your Family?* radio program was on 150 stations, at the end, over 450! And ten books that I had been working on during the last four years were all published in 1997! I believe that when one chooses to make their marriage a priority, God blesses.

An Anchor in the Time of Storm

I've spent time pondering the question, Why is it we've grown together through this crisis while others grow apart? Three things come to mind:

First, *there is no blame*. The stroke just happened! Blame is a relationship killer. It produces guilt; and guilt produces alienation. Blaming another and thus shirking personal responsibility is a terrible thing; but self-blame can be just as devastating. Saying "If only I had been there it wouldn't have happened" or "If only I had warned him" or "If only I hadn't . . ."

"If only" merely increases the pain of the crisis. If blame must be cast, let it be cast on the real culprit: sin. And let the result be a longing for a better world and a drawing closer to each other to create a little bit of heaven in this wicked world until Christ comes and puts an end to bad things.

Second, *we hold no secrets from each other*. Our words and actions travel on the solid ground of trust, not the thin ice of white lies. We aren't afraid to tell each other how we feel, to ask for what we need, to question that which we don't understand, and to honestly share that which we learn. We are in this together—united. When one hurts, the other winces; when one gains function, the other rejoices; when one gets discouraged, the other exudes hope. No play-acting here. We are one, and thus, we can be real and choose to be what the other needs. Like a mobile delicately balanced, when one part moves, the other automatically adjusts.

Third, *complete acceptance of each other is the only way of life we have ever known*. "For better or for worse; in sickness or in health . . ." is not some standard we had to work toward achieving once we suffered a crisis. It's always been the norm for our marriage. There is no need to feel self-pity or other-pity because of the stroke; no need for one to be the hero or one the victim. We're merely in this together and will each do whatever is necessary to continue to reach our adjusted goals and make our new dreams come true.

Although having a stroke is not something either of us would have chosen, we can accept what happened as reality, without denial, anger, or bitterness. *Being* together is far more important to us than *doing* things together. Acceptance of the other is 100 percent, regardless of capability, behavior, or function.

Children

Children can be another wonderful anchor in the time of storm. Yet, one should not expect them to leave their own lives behind and race to their parent's bedside, unless absolutely necessary. At the time of my stroke, our daughter, Kimberly, who lived over a thousand miles away, had a new baby and was working full time while her husband was finishing his last four months of his masters program at the University of Denver. It was not necessary, or desirable, for her to travel to Tennessee. A hospital is not a place for tiny babies. Nor was it reasonable for our son, Kevin, to drop his classes at La Sierra University in California.

But Kari, our physical therapist daughter, sensed that if her dad ever needed her, it was now. And she was right! Many times during that first five days that she stood by his side, encouraging him and making him use his reluctant muscles, Jan said to her, "I never realized that all the tuition we paid for your education would ever be needed by me!" She was a vital anchor for her dad at that moment—and for me too. She had the medical expertise Jan so desperately needed—especially since hospital physical therapy didn't start until four days after his stroke! Plus, her treatments were given with a love and concern that money can't buy!

I also sensed the need of as much of our family as possible to be involved in Jan's recovery process. I felt they needed to see him in his most helpless condition so they would appreciate the miracle of healing that we were experiencing. I also thought it would be important for them to see how determined Jan was to not let this strike get the best of him.

And so twelve days after Jan's stroke we were on the plane flying to California, where so many of our family lived. We both needed their love. We needed their hugs and their words of encouragement. For Jan, it was especially good to be with his sister, Christine, again. She always had adored him. She was Jan's second mother—always looking out for him; always putting his needs before hers. It was Chris who was attending the same college as me, who noticed I looked strikingly similar to Jan's old girlfriend and arranged a blind date! And so it was to Chris's house where we went to stay just days after Jan's stroke. As our car drove up her driveway, she came running out to meet us. Right there, Jan determined he was going to walk for his Kryszia—and he did!

Family does that for people—it brings out their best. When you're with people who believe in you, who think you're wonderful *and who accept you just the way you are*, you tend to, out of love, want to give them your best. Jan didn't have to perform for them. Their love was not built on his ability to walk, to think clearly, or to function independently. But love is powerful. And surrounded with their acceptance, Jan could risk bigger things—and thus he could grow.

But what if family turns away from you at the very time you need them the most? When crisis hits, some family members may not be able to respond with time and attention because they have their own issues they are dealing with. Don't expect too much. Don't hold it against them. Don't make them feel guilty when they can't give you what you need. You must be responsible for finding those who can give you courage and hope. Sometimes you must turn to your friends.

My family of friends

"Family" is more than flesh-and-blood bonding. Parents, grandparents, adult children, aunts, uncles, and cousins may hang together on the family tree but grow distant after months or years when they fail to invest time in each other. Divergent values can also separate. The tendency is to spend time with those who have similar interests and goals as you, those with whom you enjoy mutual respect, those with whom you feel a spiritual bond. Having the same surname doesn't ensure heart bonding and closeness. I've always mused how often family *in name only* show up at weddings or funerals— or when they're financially broke—but they seldom take the effort or spend the money to knock on your door unless they need something.

Friends, however, are wonderful gifts we give ourselves. True friends, because of shared experiences, interests, and the bonding of invested time in each other, show up for no reason at all other than to offer themselves in whatever way they can to ease your pain.

It was our incredible network of friends who kept Jan and me on the phone almost constantly once he got into his private room at Memorial Hospital. He needed that stimulation. He needed to know that in his impaired condition he was still important to them. He needed their words of encouragement and their prayers.

Our family constellation changed as we have grown older and blood relationships have scattered. We felt the change when five years before the stroke, Jan and I moved from California where we had lived for over thirty years and were surrounded by family (parents, siblings, in-laws, and children) to Tennessee where there was no immediate family.

We have found a new family in those who share time and experiences with us—and those who worship with us. Never before had I realized how important it was to have a family support network of friends.

Why is it that we are so blessed with thousands of "friends" around the world who prayed for Jan and who sent so many cards and letters that the scrapbook I put together for him is bulging at its seams? There are a couple clichés I've discovered that hold profound truth. First, "To have friends you must prove yourself friendly." And second, "You can't expect people to know if you don't tell them."

There would have been no one at the Memorial Hospital emergency room to give me support if I hadn't had the guts to let people know what was happening. Seconds after Jan had his stroke, I was on the phone. My first calls were for information; then I notified our immediate family and our family network of friends and prayer supporters. It was that family circle of friends that were at our side almost immediately.

Friends seldom just happen. Friends are made. Time must be invested, interests shared, and thoughts and feelings expressed. In short, you must become vulnerable to loss of time and effort and to misunderstandings if you want to have friends. To risk making a friend means you must risk rejection, for not everyone in this world is destined to accept your offer of friendship. When you reach out, the majority may turn their back and walk away. But unless you step forward and smile at a stranger, talk to an acquaintance, and help your neighbor, you will never discover the joy, fulfillment, and warmth of friendship.

We took the risk when we got a call from friends in Charleston, South Carolina, asking for prayer. Their plans were being dashed, and they didn't know where to turn. We had met Dianne and Oscar Kosarin a year before Jan's stroke at a "Romance at the Ranch" couples retreat in South Carolina when Jan and I were presenters and Dianne and Oscar provided the music.

There was an instant bond—especially between us two girls—and our friendship grew as couples grew. They came up to Tennessee a few times to visit us. And we went down to Charleston to see *Fiddler on the Roof*, the play for which Oscar was the musical director (he's a concert pianist) and Dianne (a concert violinist) was the "fiddler," and then we watched Oscar direct *The Christmas Carol*.

The Kosarins had planned to move to Collegedale, Tennessee (just twenty-five minutes from us), where their children could enjoy a Christian school environment. They "bought" a house, enrolled their teenage daughter in the Collegedale Academy, and arranged for her to live with another family for two months until they could make the move.

The reason for Dianne's call for prayer was that the Collegedale house was sold out from under them. One of the fine print items stated that up until the day the sale was finalized, if the sellers received a higher offer, the Kosarin's had forty-eight hours to match it. The higher offer came right before Labor Day. The Kosarin's were out of town, and by the time they got the message, it was too late to make the necessary financial arrangements—and they lost the house.

I asked Dianne if she was sure Collegedale was the place for their children to receive the Christian education they wanted. Dianne was convinced. "Then," I said, "come live with us until you find another place."

At first it may have seemed an impulsive suggestion since we had only one bedroom and a storage room for a family of four to sleep in, but I believe it was God-inspired. As it turned out, we needed them more than they needed us, even though we didn't know it at the time. It was obvious that they needed a place to stay. But we needed the laughter, the talk, the fun, and the stimulation of good friends.

Dr. Charles Thomas, Jan's friend and therapist at the Desert Hot Springs Therapy Center, had just said to him a few months before, "Jan, you need to laugh more." But when it's just the two of us and the daily routine of reading, writing, paying bills, figuring past-due taxes, and exercising reluctant muscles, there just isn't much to laugh about.

All that changed that October day when the Kosarin van pulled into our driveway with a trailer load of boxes, books, a guitar, Legos, and a pet mouse. And for three months we laughed, sang, talked far into the night, and laughed some more. Everything was funny. Dianne and I were constantly doing the same things—without consulting the other. For example, Dianne came home and announced, "I just bought a white storage cabinet, and it's in the back of my van."

"Really," I replied. "What kind?" Dianne started to describe it, and I began laughing. "I bought the same cabinet yesterday; it's still in the back of my van."

With a passion, we two women began converting the storage room into a children's bedroom. Working late into the night—or wee hours of the morning—Dianne would stop and announce, "Time for tea!" Then we would set up a box in the middle of the floor, put a towel over it, and with paint up to our elbows and speckles in our hair, we would light candles and bring out the goblets and enjoy a fruit slushie. (We have pictures to prove it!) Jan usually missed those parties—he was asleep. But the next day at dinner, he would get a complete report, and once more we'd laugh.

The house is quiet now. The Kosarin's moved into the house that was sold out from under them! Can you believe it? The house came back on the market three months later!

We miss the telephone calls for Carli—four or five per evening. We had almost forgotten the fun of being the answering service for a popular teenage girl! And we miss hearing the strum of her guitar. When Jan and I come home, we miss ten-year-old Oscar running out into the garage to greet us. Such a happy face! Children certainly brighten the dull landscape of middle age! Even now when I think back at those active evening hours with the children, I have to smile.

Isn't it interesting that God knows, so much better than we, what we need? My prayers had focused on us: "Lord, strengthen Jan's muscles; help him overcome his limp; help him have faster reaction time; help me be able to pay the bills." Let me assure you, my prayer was not "Lord, send some children to live with us." But that's what we needed most at that time in our lives.

In fact, the timing was perfect. Because at this same time our daughter, Kari, having just moved to northern Tennessee—about two and a half hours away from us—felt that Jan should stay with her and Jeff for a number of weeks so she could do some intensive therapy with him. And so it was, during the days Jan was gone, I was not alone. Not only did I have good companionship, but I found a new "sister" and prayer partner in Dianne. The Kosarin's have become family, and we are all the richer because of it.

My mind goes back to one of my favorite passages. I especially like the words from The Living Bible, "Be glad for all God is planning for you. Be patient in trouble, and prayerful always. When God's children are in need, you be the one to help them out. And get into the habit of inviting guests home for dinner or, if they need lodging, for the night" (Rom. 12:12, 13).

When the skies are blue, a gentle breeze is blowing and the seas are calm, you can get along without using an anchor. But you can't sail through life with peace of mind, unless you know it's there in case you need it. So it is with family—in whatever form "family" takes. You may go for periods of time without the need, but when the storm hits and your life becomes battered and torn, family is the anchor that helps you ride out the storm.

Taking the old familiar words of the Priscillia J. Owens' hymn "Will Your Anchor Hold" and adding "family" to the last line of the chorus, I find truth:

"We have an anchor that keeps the soul
Steadfast and sure while the billows roll;
Fastened to the Rock (Jesus Christ) which cannot move,
Grounded firm and deep in [our *family's*] love"
(Seventh-day Adventist Hymnal, 534).

CHAPTER Nine

You've Got to Have a Dream

Without a dream, life wouldn't be worth living. Since Jan's stroke, Jan's and my dreams have changed to fit the reality of our circumstances, but they are dreams just the same. Dreams are what keep hope alive. And hope is a welcome companion in tough times.

When Jan was a little boy he wanted to be rich so he could drive a car (only the rich had cars in Poland at that time), and he wanted to beat up the Nazis. He didn't like how they treated the Poles, and he was angry they took away his father.

Time passed, the war ended, the Nazi threat was gone, and his dream changed to that of his father's: to someday go to the United States of America.

Those of us who have grown up in America have no idea what this country means to those who look on from the outside but who have no visas. For Jan's family, America was the place where there were no limitations; where "money grew on trees and the streets were paved with gold."

Jan's folks never struck it rich in this country, but when Jan was seventeen they did get a car: an almost-new maroon Ford Fairlane. His father, although he never learned how to drive, could see that his family needed a car and began saving for it. It was a high day in Jan's life when he drove that car home and became the official family chauffeur. His dream had come true!

It was not until our family visited Poland in 1975 that I realized why a car meant so much to Jan as a child. But let me tell you the whole story:

In 1970, when Jan was asked to give a scientific presentation in Europe, we used our savings to get the car of his dreams from the Mercedes Benz factory in Sindelfingen, Germany.

Five years later, because of inflation, we sold that car for what we paid for it. Then because we were going back to Europe and because the first Mercedes was such a good investment, we decided to get another one and then drive into Poland to attend a statistical conference where Jan was speaking.

Let me tell you, driving a Mercedes through Communist Poland in 1975 was quite an experience. The roads sported horse-drawn wagons and a few tiny Polish- or Russian-made cars. Then around the corner would come this brand-new big, bright yellow Mercedes 240D. The people would stop and stare, and wherever we parked, crowds would gather.

In Andrahof, the little village where Jan's father had grown up, we met some people with the Kuzma surname—perhaps distant relatives—and we asked them if they would like to go for a ride and show us the sights. Can you believe it? They had never been in a passenger car before!

They took us to a resort where workers vacationed. We parked and got out to walk around. When we returned to the car there was a crowd around it. At first Jan was concerned that something had happened to the car, but then he realized that these workers had never before seen a car like this. They stroked it as if they were wooing a beautiful woman and repeated over and over, *"Takie cacko; takie cacko,"*—"Such a treasure; such a treasure."

A car was just that—a treasure—for the people of Poland. In 1975, it took a physician the equivalent of five years of full-time salary to be able to afford a car. But even if you were able to pay for one, there was such a long waiting list that it might take another year or so before your dream would come true.

When the people asked us how we got the car, Jan tried to explain (in his best Polish) that eight weeks ago he called the Mercedes dealer in California and ordered the car he wanted. He specified the color, the interior, and other special features, and then he sent them a check, and came to Germany and picked the car up at the factory. They couldn't believe it was so easy. The red tape of Poland made the process formidable, and they shook their heads in wonder.

After twenty-five years in America, Jan had grown accustomed to the good life that is so accessible here. It wasn't until that moment that he realized how very different his life would have been at forty years of age, if his father had not had the dream to come to America. He could have easily been that forty-year-old Polish Kuzma from Andrahof who had never ridden in a car, much less driven one!

Once Jan's family's dream of coming to the U.S. came true, they then dreamed of becoming citizens of this wonderful country. For five years their family studied basic American history and U.S. government, preparing for the day they would go into the Detroit courtroom, stand before the judge, renounce their previous citizenship, and swear allegiance to the United States of America.

The magic day was January 18, 1957. The day stands clearly in Jan's memory. Here's what Jan says about that experience: "Judge Frank Dingell admonished us on the privileges and possibilities of being U.S. citizens. He made us feel proud of America. He reminded us of how many people would give almost anything to be standing in our place—and we knew it was true. He told us this country was a land of opportunity, but in return it needed us to become active, responsible citizens. And I was ready to do my part by completing my education."

Jan's graduation from college was as much a fulfillment of his parents' dream for him as it was his own. They had given up their homeland, their jobs, their friends, and a cultural group who spoke their language so their children could obtain an education and take advantage of the opportunities that only the United States could offer. When Jan turned fifty-five he thought about his father coming to a foreign country at that age to literally begin again, and he wondered if he would have been so courageous.

There are many small steps that one must take in the pursuit of any dream, and so it was with Jan's dream for an education: first college, then a masters in biostatistics, and then a doctorate. At each step Jan could see the hand of God working.

One of the most memorable events he had along the way had to do with the foreign language exam required for his doctorate. Since Jan had gone to German schools as a child and lived in Germany for six years, he confidently took that exam and was the first out of hundreds to finish. The names of those who passed were posted the next day. He knew he had passed, but just to make sure, he searched the list for his name. It wasn't there.

Shocked, he asked for an explanation. Jan was told he only got 33 percent on the French test. "FRENCH?" He exclaimed. "I took the German exam!" When scored with the German key, he got nearly perfect; but he at times muses about how he got one-third of the French questions correct without knowing any French!

Most who have gone through the discipline of getting a Ph.D. have a few horror stories to tell about their qualifying exam, their research committee, or the completion of their dissertation. Jan was concerned on only two occasions.

First, there was his qualifying examination. This exam had a reputation of being extremely difficult. It covered competencies in a number of areas. Jan was most worried when he came to the question about providing a proof in mathematical statistics. He prayed when he saw that question and then breathed a sigh of relief and a prayer of thanks when he was able to solve it. Since these exams had been a stumbling block to numerous students on their journey toward their dreams, Jan prayed earnestly that God would help him pass. Four doctoral candidates sat for the exam together; three of them passed. Jan was one of the fortunate ones; and he gave the credit to God.

The next challenge had to do with the acceptance of his

dissertation proposal. After Jan's presentation, Dr. Wallace Tourtelotte, his major dissertation advisor, began to list all the other things he wanted Jan to add to his research study. He went on and on, and Jan began to break into a sweat. Finally, Dr. Dodge, another committee member, spoke up. "Dr. Tourtelotte, if Jan were to do all that you have proposed, he would be working for you for the next forty years. I think his proposal is adequate." And without much discussion, it passed.

When at last Jan had completed his doctoral requirements, he was disappointed when I learned that the University of Michigan's graduation was to be held on Sabbath. He really wanted to go. He was the first person in the history of his family to get an advanced degree. But Jan felt that God had brought him so far and had blessed him so greatly that he could not forget his weekly twenty-four-hour appointment with the Lord. Not even the promise made by the School of Public Health to give each candidate who attended graduation the expensive doctoral hoods and gowns swayed him to attend a secular event instead of "keeping the Sabbath day holy."

Jan explained to Professor Felix Moore, chairman of the Department of Biostatistics, why he could not attend the graduation ceremony. Even though Professor Moore was disappointed, he didn't try to persuade Jan otherwise.

Then a few days after graduation, Professor Moore called Jan into his office where Dr. Myron Wegman, the dean of the School of Public Health at the University of Michigan, congratulated Jan on his accomplishment. They then gave him a gown and presented him with the beautiful yellow and blue hood that symbolized his public health profession. Then they proceeded with a private graduation ceremony for Jan, including pictures. That night as Jan walked beneath the stars and looked up, he thanked God for another dream come true.

There is something interesting about dreams that shape one's life. They're not illusive; they're not "pie in the sky"; they are not bubbles that burst; they are not the wish you make upon a star. Those dreams vanish like a helium-filled balloon being carried away with a current of wind.

A dream that shapes, molds, and makes you stretch to hold it tight is an *achievable* dream. You have to see it, believe it, feel it, taste it, or you will never start your journey through the unknown to pursue its fulfillment.

Dreams that come true are not handed out on silver platters to the idle. Luck does that! And luck is reserved for the one in a billion who win the lottery or the Reader's Digest Sweepstakes.

Dreams, however, are available to all. You can't be too young to have one or too old. You can't be too sick, too disabled, or too tired. If you choose to dream, it can be yours. Dreams for most of us are what makes life worth living. And for many, they are what keeps them alive!

Yet in spite of this, some people are dream-killers. We sometimes call these mercenaries "pragmatic"; but I call them psychological murderers. They destroy hope with their inability to think beyond the here and now. Instead of words of encouragement that lift people up, they knock people down with demeaning words of criticism, sarcasm, and arguments for what they perceive as reality.

The mother who says to her child, "No one in the family has ever graduated from college. Who do you think you are, thinking you're going do it?" The father who says, "It's impossible; there's no way we are ever going to have enough money for you to do that!" The wife who says, "Run for political office? You can't even have a decent conversation with me, let alone give an intelligent speech. No one would listen to you!" The husband who says, "A woman's place is in the home. You shouldn't have had children if you wanted to do something like that." The employer who says, "I don't care if there is a better way to do it. I'm the boss, and you do what I say!" The teacher who says, "You're grades just aren't good enough."

After visiting Poland and falling in love with the soul and spirit of the people there, Jan and I began to dream of taking our children back with us for a "roots" trip. We wanted to show them the various places where he had lived as a little boy and the escape route his mother and the children had taken. The more Jan read about Polish affairs in the early months of 1986, the more a dream began to form in his mind. He wanted to have our family meet the Polish president. He wanted to discuss what we as Americans could do to enhance Polish/American relations, which were at a low ebb because of solidarity, martial law, and the economic sanctions on Poland that were imposed by the U.S.

Jan presented the idea to our daughter, Kimberly, because he thought a letter from a seventeen-year-old might have a better chance of getting through to the president's desk. She liked the idea, so together they composed a letter and addressed it to General Wojciech Jaruzelski, President, Warsaw, Poland. We had no official address.

This dream of Jan's was beyond me. I'm not a dream-killer, but I'll have to admit when I dropped the letter in the postal box, I prayed, "Lord, let this letter get lost." I couldn't, even in my wildest imagination, picture our little family, living on a five-acre grapefruit grove in Redlands, California, ever meeting with any head of a nation, let alone the Communist country of Poland.

But even if dreams sound as impossible as this one, my philosophy is to support, encourage, help, plan, and in the end celebrate! That's what a family is for!

The letter didn't get lost and on July 25, 1986, we experienced the most unlikely of all Jan's dreams coming true. It was eleven o'clock. Our family was in the Rose Room of the Belvedere Palace, which is the Polish White House. Suddenly the doors opened, and we were warmly greeted by General Wojciech Jaruzelski, the president of Poland.

We were seated around a table filled with delicacies, with Kimberly next to the general. He smiled, and his courteous and pleasant manner put us at ease!

The general thanked Kimberly for writing such a sincere letter. He then provided us with a brief history of Poland and explained that Poland was lagging in economic development because of the tremendous destruction of industry, housing, and people during World War II. The destruction of Poland was thirty-three times greater than that of Great Britain. In fact, over 85 percent of Warsaw was completely demolished!

He indicated that it was essential to impose martial law in Poland to relieve the country from anarchy, chaos, disruption of productivity, and threats to the liberty of many Polish people. What had started out being a movement of the majority of the people had become a militant religious force that no longer could be endorsed by all. If martial law had not been imposed and order restored, Russian tanks would have crossed the border and Poland would have lost the token freedom it had.

He explained what the Polish government was doing to have better relations with the workers. The solution to this situation was not an easy one, because of the attitude of hostility among the workers and the current structure of the government where the Polish government was subjected to the whims of the Russian Communist regime. Later we learned the real reason; that President Reagan was working behind the scenes with the pope to plan the demise of the Polish Communist party as the first step in bringing on the downfall of Communism.

At the time we wondered, "Why is the U.S. imposing economic sanctions on Poland when so much freedom exists there and the majority of the people approve of the government?" General Jaruzelski himself honestly expressed that trying to heal Polish/American relationships was like throwing dry peas against the wall. No matter what Poland seemed to do, it just bounced back and nothing seemed to happen.

As we stood up to leave, he embraced each of us warmly and said that he considered us to be his personal friends and hoped we could come and visit him again. Once again the doors opened and this time presents were bestowed upon us: beautiful bouquets of roses for the girls and me and then personal gifts for each of us as reminders of our trip to Poland.

When I doubt if dreams come true, I just look up on Jan's office wall and see the picture of our family standing with General Jaruzelski, and my hope is renewed. Jan has exclaimed numerous times, "Who would ever think that I, born to humble people in an apartment house in Warsaw, would fifty years later be across town in the Polish White House, talking and eating with the president!"

Dreams should never cause discouragement. A dream

should not have so much rigidity or such a tight time schedule attached to it for achievement that you cannot deal with change or delay. Dreams should not cause you to give up on the task at hand, nor should they cause you to go to the opposite extreme and become a Don Quixote, living in an illusion. A dream is something that can be visualized and wrapped in the optimistic spirit of "where there's a will, there's a way."

The safety net for achievable dreams is that one must be content enough, or accepting enough, with the present that one is not bowed down with worry, anxiety, and frustration, for these culprits steal essential brain time needed for the possibility thinking essential for figuring out options. Plus, they zap creative energy needed for pursuing the options that are considered.

What is essential is to have just enough contentment with, or acceptance of the present, to form a psychologically healthy platform from which to launch one's dreams; while at the same time a heap of hope that things will be better in the future. For it's hope that makes one willing to attempt the next seemingly "impossible" step toward making dreams come true.

I call this the "acceptance of the present with hope for the future" philosophy, the Superman Strategy. Why? Because it is seen so clearly in the life that Christopher Reeve (who is best known for his role as Superman) has been forced to live since that fateful day of May 1995. When his horse refused to jump a hurdle, he was sent hurling through the air, landing on his head and breaking his neck.

Completely paralyzed from his neck down, he can't even breathe on his own for more than an hour or two, yet he speaks of the time when medical science will know enough about his condition that he may be able to walk again. *Time* magazine (August 26, 1996, page 44) says this about Christopher, "He lies between the acceptance of the reality of his condition and the expectation of changing it. He goads the politicians to help the scientists. He goads the scientists to make him and others well. He exercises and prepares his limbs for the day when a cure might be administered. And he waits."

But even though he can't move, he doesn't wait in idleness. His interim dream is to raise awareness and funds for research to help those with spinal cord injuries. Nor does he cast blame—not even on his horse. Instead his attitude is, "It was an accident, it just happened. But now I have the opportunity to make sense out of it. I believe it's what you do *after* a disaster that gives it meaning" (ibid., 48).

Just reading about the extensive care Christopher Reeve can't live without, Jan's disabilities pale in significance. But like Christopher, Jan now has a number of personal goals that he is working hard to achieve. While Christopher is working toward being able to breathe a few minutes longer off the respirator and to clear the mucus from his lungs, Jan wants to do "wild" things like swim without his life jacket and walk without a limp. He's already learned to ride a bicycle again and play tennis. Although his tennis game isn't what it used to be, it is really quite good considering that the physicians didn't expect him to have much, if any, left-side movement. And he'd like to have the strength he once had and the energy. (Wouldn't we all?)

Jan knows what it will take to make these dreams come true: hard work and sometimes the denial of immediate gratification in order to enjoy future rewards. That's why he chose to fly out to California by himself for a month of rehabilitation at Desert Hot Springs Therapy Center. We missed each other wildly. It was the first time we had been apart since his stroke. But Jan knew he needed what Dr. Charles Thomas and his staff could give him, and I had appointments that I couldn't cancel.

Many times Jan doesn't feel like doing his exercises. Progress is so slow now that it is tempting to give up and just live with his disabilities. Just a couple weeks ago he told me, "I realize that I'm getting older, and things may never be the same." Of course, every living being is getting older, but I'm not going to let him use age as a cop-out! Instead, I find encouraging articles to read to him; facts about how others have achieved success regardless of numerous failures or advanced age.

Although Jan has always admired Abraham Lincoln, he had not realized his road to the presidency was paved with so many failures until I read him this list:

> 1816 His family was forced out of their home. He had to work to support them.
>
> 1818 His mother died.
>
> 1831 He failed in business.
>
> 1832 Ran for state legislature—lost.
>
> 1832 Also lost his job—wanted to go to law school but couldn't get in.
>
> 1833 Borrowed some money from a friend to begin a business and by the end of the year he was bankrupt. He spent the next seventeen years of his life paying off this debt.
>
> 1834 Ran for state legislature again—won.

1835 Was engaged to be married, his sweetheart died, and his heart was broken.

1836 Had a total nervous breakdown and was in bed for six months.

1838 Sought to become speaker of the state legislature—defeated.

1840 Sought to become elector—defeated.

1843 Ran for Congress—lost.

1846 Ran for Congress again—this time he won—went to Washington and did a good job.

1848 Ran for reelection to Congress—lost.

1849 Sought the job of land officer in his home state—rejected.

1854 Ran for Senate of the United States—lost.

1856 Sought the vice-presidential nomination at his party's national convention—got less than 100 votes.

1858 Ran for U.S. Senate again—again he lost.

1860 Elected president of the United States.

—Source unknown

Jan has always appreciated the philosophy voiced in Winston Churchill's famous speech, "Never, never, never give up!" And Jan is certainly not going to give up now just because he has a strike against him, even though at times he may have a fleeting feeling of regret.

Instead, we decided to invest in a place where we could enjoy being together; where I could write and where Jan could continue the water therapy that was so helpful to him. We found a little place on the beach near Cabo San Lucas, Mexico, and now our dreams have an expanded mission. The little church in San José del Cabo has no supplies for their children to learn about Jesus and enjoy the Bible stories. And wouldn't it be wonderful to have a therapy center in Mexico like Desert Hot Springs Therapy Center? So many people come to that area who need physical therapy, hydrotherapy, and massage to keep their aches and pains under control. What a witness this program could be!

Jan's new personal goal is to learn Spanish so he can communicate with the people he meets in Mexico. I'm learning too. We also want to learn as much as we can about end-time events so we can share this information with others. Every time we come to Mexico our goal is to read a new book on the subject. Our next project is to read again that classic by Ellen White, *The Great Controversy*. These are goals we didn't have before the stroke; goals that fit our interests and abilities at this time.

When bad things happen; when crisis hits, it's important to reprioritize your dreams. Dreams should never be set in cement, or they can become a millstone around your neck, pulling you down into the pits of depression when circumstances make fulfillment impossible. How much better it is to adjust that dream, remold, or change it completely and go for something equally fulfilling than to stubbornly hold on to an inflexible dream and become discouraged when, regardless of how hard you work, it's just not going to happen. Just never give up a dream unless you replace it with another. Without a dream, you will slowly die and eventually perish.

The best dreams, and those that are ultimately most fulfilling, are those that you hold in tandem with God. Don't be afraid to give your dream to God and pray that God will reveal whether or not the dream is one He has for you or whether it is merely a selfish one of your own. How will you know? The answer is to keep moving forward. If you're standing still, you'll never know if the next door will be open or closed. If it's closed, reprioritize or find an alternative route. If it's open, go for it!

When I'm tempted to think "It's impossible," I have a number of "dream" texts that encourage me. My favorite is:

> Delight yourself also in the Lord,
> And He shall give you the desires of your heart.
> Commit your way to the Lord,
> Trust also in Him,
> And He shall bring it to pass
> (Ps. 37:4, 5, NKJV).

Living by this philosophy can keep you from discouragement when the wait seems exceptionally long or when you're tempted to give up.

Change Is
Never Easy

During those first twenty-four hours after Jan's stroke, I encountered the sympathy of many. The emergency room doctor, "I'm so sorry this happened to you." The cardiologist, "It's dense. I'm so very sorry." The neurologist, "I'm sorry to have to tell you this, but the stroke was massive." Everyone shook their heads in disbelief that such a thing could have happened. It was a terrible thing. But their pity didn't give me hope. Their sympathy, although well-meaning, just reinforced the miserable plight we were in. If I had any thoughts of "poor me," their expressions of concern just dug the pit a little deeper.

Later Jan expressed his feelings like this, "I know people feel sorry for me. If I were them, I'd feel sorry for me too. Even if I were a vindictive person with a bitter enemy, a stroke is a curse I wouldn't wish on anyone. But I don't need their pity; I need their hope. I don't need to mourn what I've lost; I need to be thankful about what I have left. I need to be encouraged that change, no matter how difficult, can be good for a person. This is a road I've never had to travel before. I need to know the journey can be a pleasant and exciting one."

A wound can be cleaned, bound up, and in time it will heal. A tumor can be cut out and, if it hasn't spread, the prognosis can be fairly good. But in either case, you basically don't change. You think the same; your personality is the same. There is no such assurance with a stroke. Because a stroke destroys your brain—the master control system of your body— the damage is pervasive.

A stroke, depending upon the location of the strike and its severity, can change everything about you: your body functions, your energy level, your personality, your speech, and your ability to move, to analyze, to plan, and to execute actions. Everything! In one awful moment one can be tumbled from the height of functionality and productivity and rendered maimed, disabled, and in some cases paralyzed.

Every disease has its challenges. Some come on slowly and you live knowing that unless God intervenes or you get a needed transplant, you must learn to cope with progressive disability and pain and in the end (after all the suffering) you'll die. Other diseases come crashing down on you like cancer, heart disease, and stroke.

Cancer is a cruel, painful, and frightening killer, but there is either an expected cure with a prescribed treatment (which may in itself cause more suffering than the cancer), or there's a projected course to the disease, and you accept the inevitable. There are many things that may affect the outcome: your diet, your attitude, and your medication. But when you've got cancer you pretty much know what you have. Only brain cancer destroys the real you—your personality.

Heart disease can be a sudden killer, but more generally it means clogged arteries, a heart attack—or a threatened one— a radical change in diet and lifestyle to prevent further problems, or as a last resort, bypass surgery. If you have advanced heart disease where blood is not being pumped efficiently to the brain, your thinking processes may be slowed, but your control panel is still intact.

But a stroke attacks the center of your being—your master control system. When nerve connections have been knocked out, everything else is affected, like ripples in a lake.

Having a stroke is like having your computer hard drive crash. Data is scrambled or inaccessible. Some information may be lost permanently. Certain functions no longer work. But unlike a computer, you can't just install a new hard drive! They don't do brain transplants!

Destroyed brain cells can't be resurrected. But your brain, unlike a hard drive, does have the amazing power to reprogram itself. You can rebuild. That's what Jan's in the process of doing with good nutrition, exercise, and a positive attitude. And we're all encouraged with his progress—but it's slow.

If a lost function is performed over and over again, new pathways can be formed in the brain. Dr. Elden Chalmers, our clinical psychologist friend, explained it to us. Every time you focus your effort to perform a function that was once automatic—even though part of the brain's nerve system that performed that function may be destroyed or substantial amounts of wiring may be lost because of the stroke—your brain will sprout new connections to restore the function.

If part of the needed brain center is not destroyed, sometimes the brain instructs the remaining portion to carry the entire load. If the required parts are completely destroyed by the stroke, the brain will figure out new wiring to perform the function. In any case, the secret is persevering, focused effort. Do it enough and eventually a new connection will be made.

The problem with most stroke patients is that they work hard for the first few months after the stroke, and then when insurance no longer pays or they cease to see much progress, they become discouraged and quit. If their eyes could just look at what is happening in their brains and if they would realize how close they were to making a connection, they would most certainly continue the hard work of rehabilitation until the connection is made. But they give up too soon and never regain the movement or function.

You would have had to know Jan before his stroke to understand the extent of the damage it has caused in his life. He feels like the same person, he has the same memories and dreams. But there is so much about him that is different. Sometimes he feels he needs to introduce himself again. If so, he'd say something like this: "My given name is spelled 'J-a-n,' pronounced 'Yon.' As a boy they called me Janek, pronounced 'Yonic.' When I came to the United States, no one knew how to pronounce my European name so I became Jan, as in January, to all except a few academic colleagues of European descent. Now since my stroke, I find myself reverting to my given name. When people ask, I tell them 'My name is 'Yon.' "

Why am I telling you this? Because Jan himself realizes that he's not the same person he was before the stroke, and his way of symbolizing a change of his identity is by adopting the original pronunciation of his name.

In many ways he is no longer the Jan I married and lived with for almost thirty-five years. He is rebuilding himself— reprogramming his "hard drive" patterned after the person he was, but it will probably never be the same. Perhaps it will help you bridge the gulf from what was, to what is, if you see my husband as "Yon." A new name designating a new stage and direction in his life, as was so often given in Bible times as, for example, Abram became Abraham or Jacob became Israel.

If you were Jan's friend before, it must have been, at least partially, because of who he was then. I wonder, will you still be drawn to the person Jan is now or the person he is in the process of becoming? To "Yon" instead of Jan?

Maybe you enjoyed good, stimulating conversation, quick comebacks, clever sayings, facts gleaned from current events, keen economic savvy, or a thoughtful analysis of political trends. He's not the critic, the analyst, and the commentator he used to be. Now he's the listener. He may think of something while you're talking, but often by the time he gets around to saying it, you have either hung up the phone or have moved on to another topic. Will you still want to be his friend when you have to carry the conversation? Will you still want to talk with him when there are long periods of silence or his response is inappropriate to the immediate topic? He's making incredible progress in this area, but he still has a long way to go.

Maybe you enjoyed planning projects with him. Was it the new ideas, the innovative approaches, or the sense of accomplishment you enjoyed when you were together? Perhaps you appreciated his optimistic "nothing's impossible" philosophy. Since the stroke, he finds himself relying a lot more on the Lord rather than his own ability to get things done. That's good!

Maybe you admired his independent spirit. He never was threatened when others chose the broad road; he didn't mind walking alone down the path less traveled. He didn't need others to applaud him. He could stand alone, if he were standing on principle. He no longer has an independent spirit. No longer does he want to chart and analyze unknown risky jungle trails of business, finance, or even church politics. He doesn't even want to take a plane to California by himself, even though he's done it. He's grown dependent. I wonder, will you still want to be around him when he may need to lean on you, rather than Jan being someone on whom you can lean?

Maybe you felt secure when you were together because you knew Jan, like Indiana Jones, could always figure out what to do next. He can't do that now. He can't even figure out how to stop a leak in the kitchen sink, let alone keep the checkbook balanced. He even has trouble getting the right telephone number when he's sure he has dialed correctly.

Maybe you liked his type A way of getting things done. Perhaps you enjoyed being on committees with Jan because he would move the agenda along: making motions, calling "question," and anticipating the need for a second. He was a born administrator. He could rally the troops; he could see what needed to be done and was not afraid to do the task or assign others the job.

If that dynamic "I Can" spirit was what you liked, will you like his new double type B personality? Will it bother you to see him doing nothing when he could be doing everything? He can now let the world go by without feeling he has to push it. Are you willing to sit back with him and just let things happen, rather than having to be in the thick of the action? If you liked his type A personality where life was lived in the fast lane, will you find his double type B one frustrating or boring?

I've often thought how scary it must be to Jan to be starting out life at sixty years of age with a new personality. Most changes of personality, at least after adulthood, are planned and come over a period of time. You decide you're going to be more assertive or more contemplative, more disciplined or more relaxed. And you set out to practice that which you would like to become, until having practiced it enough these behaviors become absorbed into your being.

The changes to Jan's personality happened instantaneously on February 8 at 7:20 p.m. He had no choice about the change. One moment he was Jan Kuzma the doer. And the next Jan Kuzma the nondoer! I like to say he went from being a human "doing" to a human "being"!

He spends a lot of time now just being. When our son, Kevin, a classic type B while growing up, used to sit and just stare out the window daydreaming, it always bothered Jan's type A personality. What a waste of time! He never could let the kids just watch TV. They had to be doing something productive as they watched. Now Jan's the person he never wanted his children to become.

Here's just one illustration of what I mean. One day about six months after the stroke, Jan and I were leisurely walking along the beach. After that, we swam in the pool and then I said I was going back inside to write. Jan replied, "I'll be along shortly, I just want to sit in the jacuzzi for a while."

He turned the control knob for the air bubbles to thirty minutes and began to soak, enjoying the pleasure of the warm water and the solitude with God. An hour later, I got worried and came down to check on him. He was still soaking, looking out across the sand into the ceaseless rolling waves. He had no idea the timer had broken. He had no idea of the passage of time. He was enjoying himself, thinking, planning, praying, counting the waves. He may have sat there all day, if I had not reminded him of the time!

Later as he was sitting in his wet bathing suit on the lounge chair putting on his sandals, fully intending to go in for lunch, he looked up and was particularly struck with the ferocious beauty of the angry white-capped waves driven by a strong ocean wind. He was mesmerized. He watched wave after wave, sometimes he could count up to seven white-capped swells coming in at once. He sat there for another twenty minutes or so, absorbed in the rhythm, the sound, and the constancy of the never-ending waves, until I once more brought him back to reality, "Are you hungry?" I asked. I don't know if Jan had ever, before the stroke, really taken the time to be one with nature.

There are many things that are very positive about the person Jan is now. One of the most healthy is probably that he is no longer driven by time. The stroke knocked out his internal clock. But to me, who married a man who lived by that clock, it's tough to adjust. I now am the one who says, "Honey, we have to leave in ten minutes, you must put your shoes on." I'm the one who struggles to keep meals served at somewhere near a regular time. I'm the one who sees that "it's past midnight, and we really must get to bed!"

The stroke also damaged Jan's initiation response. It's difficult for him to move with purpose, focus on what needs to be done, and do it. I'm the one who now says, "Sweetheart, you've been watching TV for two hours, you need to get up and exercise." I'm the one who has a difficult time watching him stand waist deep in the cool swimming pool for fifteen or twenty minutes without getting in and swimming. I can't believe I've become a pushy person, but I have!

Jan used to be able to do many things at once. Not anymore. He can't focus on two things at once. If I'm talking to him on the phone and something interesting happens next to him, I have to wait until I can again capture his attention. He can't watch TV and do anything else, not even exercise. It's typical of the Attention Deficient Disorder we see in children. And just like an ADD child, it doesn't bother him, but it sure can be annoying to the people living with him! But it's getting better. Those nerve endings are growing. Connections are being made. There's hope!

As I stop to analyze Jan's life now, it's not just the effects of the stroke that have left him changed forever. I'm sure it's also the high doses of Coumidin that zap his energy. He doesn't like having to be dependent on medication. He doesn't like the way it makes him feel; but I can assure you, neither of us like the alternative either, that of taking the risk that his heart will throw another clot. So he will take the lesser of two evils for the rest of his life—caught in the riptide of "you're damned if you do and damned if you don't."

That leaves Jan—and me—with two choices about how we should live: Either we resist the change and merely exist through a life we never wanted or planned, or we accept the fact that Jan has changed, and is continuing to change, and enjoy the adventure of what life now has in store for us. We choose the second option. And we invite you to come along.

Life is dynamic. It moves. It ebbs and flows like the tide.

Good friends ebb and flow together. As one grows, the other stretches; as one retreats, the other adjusts. Life goes on. Years change things. We all grow old.

I do not object to natural forces nudging us along; change little by little can be adjusted to. I have no doubt that, together, friends can change and lose nothing but gain everything in a growing relationship. Becoming something new; developing ourselves would be mentally stimulating and psychologically healthy.

But it is natural for people who have experienced a dramatic change in their lives, as Jan has done, to fear that the change has been too abrupt for some, too dramatic for their family and friends to adjust to. The result is that, instead of accepting the change and enjoying the challenge of the new relationship, they push the person into trying to become the person they once were.

A stroke victim has no choice in the matter. So the choice is ours. Will we choose to accept these individuals just the way they are, or will we go our own way and find relationships that better meet our own needs? The sad fact is that when accident or illness causes personality changes, friendships and marriages sometimes break up. And to add to the pain, it's usually when both need each other the most!

People going through change don't want you to feel sorry for them, even though it's quite natural to do so. They don't need your pity. That will only make them feel sorry for themselves and keep them from accepting who they are now. It's in accepting themselves, with all their skills and disabilities, that they can be most healthy psychologically.

One cannot hold on to too much of life at once. If one holds too tightly to the past, one cannot reach for the opportunities that only the future can hold. Like the monkey with his hand stuck in the cookie jar because he won't let go of what he's got, you can't take hold of the new without releasing the old. Don't hold on to the memories of who your friend, family member, or mate used to be so tightly that you can't accept who they are now. I challenge you to jump across the gap and enjoy the adventure. That's what I'm doing, and Jan and I are enjoying our new relationship.

I have always loved him; and I always will. I liked the old Jan, but I like the new one too. What's really important is that we have each other.

But not all of the old Jan has changed. As I consider his life there are two areas, no three, that haven't changed.

The first is his "dry" sense of humor. He never lost that. By the second day after his stroke, he was coming up with so many clever comments that Kari started writing them down. For example, when he learned that Jeff, Kari's husband, was going on a dirt bike ride, and knowing how Jeff sometimes pushed the limits for the thrill of the ride, Jan said, "I don't mind sharing my hospital room with Jeff, but I hope he doesn't get hurt."

When my sister, Dianne, and her husband, Gary, brought Jan some grapes, he asked with a twinkle in his eye, "Are those grapes from Canaan?"

Kari started to give him a drink and accidentally spilled some as she made the comment, "Here's some water you can drink." Her dad came back with, "Or take a shower."

After reading about how Abram's wife Sarai, when she got pregnant at ninety years of age, was referred to as a wrinkled prune in Max Lucado's book, *Applause of Heaven*, I asked Jan if he wanted anything more to eat for breakfast. He replied, "I'll take some Sarai fruit." I didn't understand at first, until he explained, "I'd like a wrinkled prune."

The second area that hasn't changed is Jan's devotional and prayer life. He still enjoys his morning time alone where he reads his Bible and the morning devotional for the day and prays. He still spends a lot of time in prayer. Kneeling is more difficult now, but if you find him sitting still with his eyes closed, he's not always dozing, although he does that a lot too. He's very likely praying. Jan says, "I believe in intercessory prayer. Just because I've had a stroke and can't do many of the things I used to do doesn't mean I can't make an impact upon my world. My best tool is prayer, and I use it often."

"I can't thank God enough for sparing my life and sparing me the devastation that was predicted during the first twenty-four hours after my stroke. God is so good, so powerful, so loving. Spontaneously, my heart erupts in praise; my thoughts voice the psalmist's words,

> Bless the Lord, O my soul: and all that is within me, bless his holy name.
>
> Bless the Lord, O my soul, and forget not all his benefits:
>
> Who forgiveth all thine iniquities; who healeth all thy diseases;
>
> Who redeemeth thy life from destruction; who crowneth thee with loving kindness and tender mercies;
>
> Who satisfieth thy mouth with good things; so that thy youth is renewed like the eagle's (Ps. 103:1-5, KJV).

I have so much to be thankful for!"

Jan also has a prayer list. Heading his list are the names of our children. We usually pray together for our children as we walk around the circular drive in front of our home. Jan prays for each, specifically, depending upon what their circumstances are and his perception of their needs.

But most of all he pleads for their salvation. They are so precious to both of us. We love them so much. And we don't think we have much more time left in this old world. We're convinced that there is nothing more important than doing the will of God and being ready for His coming. We sense this urgency, but we realize our age and Jan's condition has something to do with where our priorities are.

Our children, however, are right now at the peak of their physical prowess, just starting exciting careers and having families. We realize it's not common to yearn for heaven when your present existence is very close to "heaven on earth." We want for them the very best of this world; yet we want them to long for heaven. We sometimes wonder if this is an oxymoron. And so Jan prays for them many times a day.

And he prays for me. He tells me often how precious I am to him. He says if it were not for my energy, my creativity, my planning, and my determination to find the good life regardless of what may happen to either of us, he doesn't know what would have happened to him. So he prays for me, not just because he needs me but more so because he loves me and wants God's blessings to be abundantly poured out on me.

He also reminds me that he prays for me because others need me. He prays for Family Matters, my organization to help families. He prays for my speaking appointments, my radio program, and my writing assignments. He prays for me as I counsel parents who need insight into family problems.

He asks that God will give me Holy Spirit wisdom to know what to say to help them find solutions. I know that he wishes he could do more to physically lighten my load, but that's impossible now, and so he knocks on heaven's door in my behalf.

And Jan prays for others. His list of those who need intercessory prayer is longer now because he is more aware of those suffering from injustice or with disease, disability, and discouragement.

There's more. He prays for our church, it's pastors, and leaders. He's interested in the welfare of Christian education and health institutions and asks God to bless. He's concerned about world governments, political injustice, war, violence, and crime, and he tells God about it.

Why does Jan pray? Because he knows it makes a difference. And he wants his life to count for something. He wants to make a difference in the world in which he lives.

There's one more thing that hasn't changed since the stroke, and for which I am most thankful. Jan and I still enjoy our intimate times together. We are as much one as we ever were. In fact, our marriage bonds have strengthened since the stroke. Before, we could go our own ways and survive fairly well. Now, Jan knows he needs me to help keep his life organized; to take care of the thousands of little details that Jan no longer thinks about or has the energy or ability to take care of. And I need him for love and companionship. I tell Jan over and over, *"Love and relationship are more important than function and productivity."* I think he is beginning to believe I mean it!

In an article I wrote shortly after the stroke, I said it this way: "It would be nice if Jan could drive, ride a bicycle, swim, and walk without a limp. It would be nice if I could produce radio scripts and columns as quickly as I did before I carried the workload of two. It would be nice—but it's not necessary. What is important is our love and relationship. We do everything together now since he needs me to get him where he needs to go and make sure things are organized. So we have more time to talk, and our marriage has never been stronger."

Change is never easy. Sudden change is even more difficult. Changing so quickly, so drastically, can so easily throw a relationship out of balance. But if Jan can accept the change in himself and not pine away for what used to be or what could have been, and if I can accept the change, then we're confident that others will.

Perhaps Jan's change is most difficult for our children, who must now adjust to a role reversal in their relationship with him. Where he was once the one who was telling them what to do, how and when, and looking out for their welfare, now they are taking care of him and reminding him of what he needs to do! As much as a young person might resist fatherly advice and wish for independence, when the father they have known all their lives is no more and will never be the same again, they, too, must grieve.

But I hope not for long, for the person Jan is now may be more what they were wishing for during their teen years when they needed their independence and he was reluctant to grant it. Jan's a much better listener now. He's much more hesitant to make suggestions because he realizes he might not perceive things as clearly as he once thought he did. And now he has time. Time literally has no meaning for him. He eats when he gets up and gets around to it. His schedule is flexible. If he feels like sleeping, he sleeps. He has time now to just be with his children: time to talk, play, listen, or do nothing. I think the new Jan will make a good grandfather.

We have found that we can survive crises; we can adjust to major change. I believe it has made us stronger individuals and stronger marriage partners.

Because Jan used to take care of so many things like property, finances, taxes, investments, and home maintenance, I used to tell Jan, "I don't know what I'd do if something terrible happened to you." Now I know. I would survive.

I know it hurts Jan that he can't help shoulder more of my burdens and responsibilities as was his custom. But that's life. He must keep telling himself that his job is to be my emotional support right now, rather than my physical support. And the change has probably been good for both of us.

But most of all, we have learned that one strike against you doesn't mean you're out. There are blessings at midnight. You *can* adjust to change. Change is never easy, but there is a sense of excitement in facing the unknown, making decisions, and having new experiences.

Our prayer is . . .

> "God grant me the serenity to accept the things I cannot change,
>> courage to change the things I can,
>> and wisdom to know the difference."

Get Up and Win Your Race

Do you have a strike against you? Most people do! But one, two, or even three strikes doesn't have to mean you're out. In God's game of life, you're never out. You have an incredible built-in ability to regenerate or recreate. God designed you that way. You can experience healing, whether your strike is physical, mental, emotional, relational, spiritual, or financial. You can find fulfillment, satisfaction, and success if you choose to do so.

The battles of your life are won or lost in your mind. Psychologically, you have the ability to fight on if you believe you can. I've been spurred on by James M. Barrie's old Scottish ballad,

> "Fight on, my men, said Sir Andrew Barton,
> I am somewhat hurt, but am not slaine,
> I'll lie me down and bleed awhile.

And then I'll rise and fight againe."
(From: Harry Moyle Tippett, *Who Waits in Faith*,
Review and Herald Publishing Association, 1951.)

This can be your experience. You may have to "lie me down and bleed awhile," but the important thing is that you will yourself to "rise and fight againe." The strength of your will can accomplish incredible things.

Victor Frankl once said, "Everything can be taken from a man but one thing: the last of the human freedoms—to choose one's attitude in any given set of circumstances, to choose one's own way" (Victor E. Frankl, *Man's Search for Meaning* [N.Y.: Pocket Books, 1963], 104).

One of my favorite poems is by T. C. Hamlet about two frogs and the choice they made after finding themselves in a can of cream. Here's how it goes:

> Two frogs fell into a can of cream
> Or so I've heard it told;
> The sides of the can were shiny and steep,
> The cream was deep and cold.
> "O, what's the use?" croaked Number 1.
> " 'Tis fate; no help's around.
> Goodbye, my friends! Goodbye, sad world!"
> And weeping still, he drowned.
> But Number 2, of sterner stuff,
> Dog-paddled in surprise,
> The while he wiped his creamy face
> And dried his creamy eyes.
> "I'll swim awhile, at least," he said—
> Or so I've heard it said;

"It really wouldn't help the world
If one more frog were dead."
An hour or two he kicked and swam,
Not once he stopped to mutter,
But kicked and kicked and swam and kicked,
Then hopped out, via butter!
—*Author Unknown*

I don't know what your "can of cream" may be! But I do know that all things are possible if you don't give up. In the worst of my hard times I've reread James 1:2-4 (NKJV) and pondered the message. "My brethren, count it all joy when you fall into various trials, knowing that the testing of your faith produces patience. But let patience have its perfect work, that you may be perfect and complete, lacking nothing."

The Living Bible puts it this way: "Dear brothers, is your life full of difficulties and temptations? Then be happy, for when the way is rough, your patience has a chance to grow. So let it grow, and don't try to squirm out of your problems. For when your patience is finally in full bloom, then you will be ready for anything, strong in character, full and complete."

And isn't that the ultimate goal in life? To be strong in character, full and complete? To me that is success.

You may have been born with a strike against you, a physical or mental defect that makes life more challenging. Or an accident may have maimed you.

As the years have gone by you may have experienced rejection by family or friends, or you may still be plagued by dyslexia or Attention Deficit Disorder, which has made academic success an illusive dream.

You may right now find yourself in a hospital bed, tied to tubes, fighting pain, and facing an unknown future; or perhaps you're home now, weak, frightened, and alone. Losing your health is a cruel strike to overcome, and it takes hard work and perhaps a lifestyle change to rebuild it. But even accepting the fact that you will eventually die doesn't have to mean you are defeated, if you continue to live with hope, honor, dignity, and integrity.

Your loss might be financial. Perhaps your job was terminated, and now that you're nearing retirement age, the hope of finding another is pretty slim. Or you may have been sued, and the judgment went against you, stealing away your savings and your children's inheritance.

Your strike might be the loss of a baby—too tiny to breathe on its own—a baby that already held all your hopes and dreams for the future. Or perhaps you lost that child grown tall, in a freak motorcycle, hiking, or water-skiing accident.

The loss of a spouse ranks at the top of life's stress-related incidents. Divorce means feelings of failure, regret, and rejection. Death rips away security, companionship, and years of accumulated dreams. Gone! Life will never again be the same.

Your loss may have been inflicted upon you in childhood through neglect or abuse, leaving a residue of unresolved issues, pain, and rejection.

Your strike may be unfair gossip or a false accusation that shreds your reputation and you stand by helplessly as those you thought to be friends fall away like flies.

But regardless of what the strike against you is, you don't have to drown in discouragement. You don't have to roll over like a wounded possum and give up. You don't have to spend the rest of the game sitting on the bench feeling like a miserable failure.

I learned a valuable lesson about success from Peter Nelson, a forty-five-year-old dentist from San Luis Obispo, who was asked to join the 1991 United States South Polar Route Expedition to climb Mt. Everest, the highest mountain in the world (29,028 feet). It was very unusual for a man his age, who was not a professional climber, to be asked to join the ten-member team, but his healthy vegetarian lifestyle made him one of the strongest.

The team started the climb at the end of the road in a little place called Jeri. From there to base camp was a two-week trip covering 120 miles; up 36,000 feet and down 24,000 feet. I often think of that trip, with a sixty-pound pack on your back, as characteristic of life in this world—constantly filled with ups and downs and burdens to be carried.

Imagine the effort it took just to get to base camp at 17,500 feet where you began the actual ascent! Just to get to base camp there were 263 porters and 15 Tibetan Sherpas (guides) needed to carry the food and supplies!

The next task was to climb Kumbu Ice Falls, a 2,000-foot climb to camp 2 at 19,500 feet, in minus 10-degree weather over a constantly shifting ice pack. Sometimes the climbers had to cross crevasses sixteen to eighteen feet across, latching together ladders and holding onto a tiny rope as they gingerly made their way across the slippery rungs of the ladder with their heavy boots and crampons. The climb was strenuous! They ate six thousand to seven thousand calories a day and still lost weight!

After reaching camp 2, the climbers put down their sixty-pound packs and hiked back down to base camp, picked up another pack, and headed over those treacherous ice falls two more times, carrying the supplies they needed.

Then it was on to camp 3, again making three trips and then finally up to camp 4, which was at an elevation of 27,000 feet—just 2,000 feet from the top. If you could get to camp 4 and the weather was clear, you would almost certainly make it to the top—to success!

From camp 3 to camp 4 took 6 hours of hard climbing. The weather was clear as the first members of the team left camp 3. What they needed most was someone with the stamina to break the way for the rest of them—like the lead goose breaks the wind for the others. Peter Nelson was chosen for the task. He pushed himself to make the 5,000 foot climb to camp 4 in one day, hoping that the next day his team could successfully finish the 2,000 foot climb to the top.

As he was coming into camp 4 with two professional climbers who were both fifteen years younger than he, he began feeling his lungs fill up with fluid. He had pulmonary edema—altitude sickness. Many get it at fourteen thousand to fifteen thousand feet, and you can die in twenty to forty minutes. The only remedy is to get to a lower altitude so the fluid goes back into the blood system. But hiking back down the mountain in the dark was suicide. His only choice was to sit up all night, breathing oxygen, praying to live until morning to have the chance to make it back down to camp 2 where they had a "Gamoff Bag" that he could be zipped into and the pressure lowered to the equivalent of six thousand to eight thousand feet.

He lived through the night and as a perfect climbing day dawned, he said Goodbye to his teammates, certain of their success in reaching the top, while he began his climb down the mountain in an attempt to save his life.

He survived, even though many that summer died on the mountain. And his team made it safely to the top.

What makes a person keep going when things get tough? For Peter it was the word *aspire*, which was the motto for the team. Here is the poem that kept him pushing forward when his muscles ached and he thought he couldn't take another step:

Aspire
"Lord, let me not be too content
With life in trifling service spent
Make me aspire!
When days with petty cares are filled
Let me with fleeting thoughts be filled
With something higher."
—*Author Unknown*

There are many lessons one can learn from climbers who have successfully scaled the tallest peaks on earth, but I think the most important for me was what Peter said about success. When he was asked how he felt having failed to reach the top, Peter replied, "Success is in running the race. I had an opportunity to climb Mt. Everest. Reaching the top would have been wonderful, but what's really important is that you climb all the mountains in your life with courage and joy."

The second lesson was in the form of a letter that was waiting for him at base camp. Peter's mother had written it weeks before, not knowing whether he would successfully reach the top or not. It simply said:

Think big
Talk small
Love much
Laugh easily
Work happily
Play fair
Give cheerfully
Receive gratefully
Thank God
And be kind!

I think the reason so many give up when they have a strike against them is that they have the wrong definition of success. If success for you is always hitting the ball, always winning the game, always reaching the top, you are destined for discouragement.

Life isn't like that. No one wins at everything. There's no such thing as a perfect ten in living.

We all make mistakes; bad things happen to good people; tragedy hits the faithful and unjust alike. There's no insurance policy to protect you from having a strike against you.

But if you see success as an attitude of courage and joy to continue playing the game of life, regardless of the strikes against you, you will have lived successfully. Jan has a strike against him, but he's not going to let discouragement blow him off the mountain!

Jesus didn't.

If there was ever a person who could have been discouraged and given up, it was Jesus. Born into poverty to a woman who got pregnant before she was married, raised with jealous stepsiblings, and stoned by His hometown friends and neighbors! That would be enough to cripple most. But not Jesus. He carried on the work His Father had given Him, getting up each time He was pushed down, even though He had no assurance of where the next meal was coming from or where He would lay His head. He was essentially a Galilean street person! He had no academic degrees, wrote no books, and had no VIPs to fund His mission. And as for His followers? They could easily have been voted most unlikely to succeed. Yet, because of their faith in Jesus, they turned the world upside down.

Can you imagine how hard it must have been for Jesus, knowing He was facing in the next few hours the most painful, cruel death possible, to say to His Father, "Thy will be done"! He said it, but He never gave up! To the very end with all the strikes of the world against Him, He continued His Father's work, even witnessing to the thief while he was hanging on the cross!

The question is, will you say "Thy will be done" and keep going? Will you accept the fact that you have a strike against you, and at the same time resolve that you'll not let it get you down? Regardless of how many times you fall and feel like a failure, will you get up and continue running the race God has for you to run?

Will you resolve to say with David,

> As for me, I will call upon God,
> And the Lord shall save me.
> Evening and morning and at noon
> I will pray, and cry aloud,
> And He shall hear my voice.
> He has redeemed my soul in peace

from the battle which was against me
(Ps. 55:16-18, NKJV).

And then will you "Cast your burden on the Lord"? His promise is that "He shall sustain you" (Ps. 55:22).

One strike doesn't mean you're out! When Jan had his stroke and I felt the world we had known was crumbling, I came across a poem that brings tears to my eyes and hope to my heart every time I read it.I pray it will instill within you the hope you need to rise each time you fall.

The Race

"Quit!" "Give up, you're beaten," they shout and plead,
there's just too much against you now, this time you can't succeed.
And as I start to hang my head in front of failure's face,
my downward fall is broken by the memory of a race.
And hope refills my weakened will as I recall that scene,
for just the thought of that short race rejuvenates my being.

A children's race, young boys, young men; how I remember well,
excitement sure, but also fear, it wasn't hard to tell.
They all lined up so full of hope, each thought to win that race
or tie for first, or if not that, at least take second place.
Their fathers watched from off the side, each cheering for his son,
and each boy hoped to show his dad that he would be the one.

The whistle blew and off they went, young hearts and hopes of fire,
to win, to be the hero there, was each young boy's desire.
One boy in particular, his dad was in the crowd,
was running near the lead and thought "My dad will be so proud."
But as he speeded down the field across a shallow dip,

the little boy who thought to win, lost his step and slipped.
Trying hard to catch himself, his hands, flew out to brace,
and mid the laughter of the crowd he fell flat on his face.

So, down he fell and with him hope, he couldn't win it now.
Embarrassed, sad, he only wished to disappear somehow.
But as he fell his dad stood up and showed his anxious face,
which to the boy so clearly said, "Get up and win that race!"
He quickly rose, no damage done, behind a bit that's all,
and ran with all his mind and might to make up for his fall.
So anxious to restore himself, to catch up and to win,
his mind went faster than his legs, he slipped and fell again.

He wished that he had quit before with only one disgrace.
I'm hopeless as a runner now, I shouldn't try to race.
But, in the laughing crowd he searched and found his father's face,
that steady look that said again, "Get up and win that race!"
So he jumped up to try again, ten yards behind the last,
if I'm to gain those yards, he thought, I've got to run real fast.
Exceeding everything he had, he regained eight or ten,
but trying so hard to catch the lead, he slipped and fell again.

Defeat! He lay there silently, a tear dropped from his eye,
there's no sense running anymore—three strikes, I'm out—why try.
The will to rise had disappeared, all hope had fled away,
so far behind, so error prone, closer all the way.
"I've lost, so what's the use," he thought, "I'll live with my disgrace."
But then he thought about his dad, who soon he'd have to face.
"Get up," an echo sounded low. "Get up and take your place.
You were not meant for failure here, get up and win that race."
With borrowed will, "Get up," it said, "you haven't lost at all,

Get Up and Win Your Race

for winning's not more than this to rise each time you fall."

So up he rose to run once more, and with a new commit,
he resolved that win or lose, at least he wouldn't quit.
So far behind the others now, the most he'd ever been,
still he gave it all he had and ran as though to win.
Three times he'd fallen stumbling, three times he rose again.
Too far behind to hope to win, he still ran to the end.

They cheered the winning runner as he crossed, first place;
head high and proud and happy—no falling, no disgrace.
But, when the fallen youngster crossed the line, last place,
the crowd gave him the greater cheer for finishing the race.
And even though he came in last with head bowed low, unproud,
you would have thought he'd won the race, to listen to the crowd.
And to his dad he sadly said, "I didn't do so well."
"To me, you won," his father said, "You rose each time you fell."

And now when things seem dark and hard and difficult to face,
the memory of that little boy helps me in my own race.
For all of life is like that race, with ups and downs and all.
And all you have to do to win is rise each time you fall.
"Quit!" "Give up, you're beaten," they still shout in my face,
but another voice within me says, "Get up and win that race."

—Author Unknown (From: *In Praise of Children*, Kay Kuzma, editor, Review and Herald Publishing Association, 1997.)

Epilogue
by Jan W. Kuzma

It's been two years since my stroke.

It would be wonderful to be able to say God has restored me completely. Yet after all, I did have a devastating stroke. But the Lord isn't finished with me yet, and I'm not giving up. Each day I work on improving the functions that were impaired. Kari, my physical-therapist daughter, is constantly coming up with new exercises, and Kay says she's seeing improvement. That's encouraging!

My reaction time is faster, and I feel great!

I've finished the revision of my biostatistics textbook and am pretty much handling our family's finances once again.

The best news, I am now driving! Do you know what that means to a man?

God has sustained us through a very difficult time and has given us the good life, in spite of the bad.

I am a living testimony that even though that thief, the devil, tried to steal my happiness, kill my ability to function, and destroy our lives, Jesus has given life back to us, even more abundantly!